Elvan Kut

**Neurochemical Aspects of Emotional Pain Modulation**

Elvan Kut

# Neurochemical Aspects of Emotional Pain Modulation

## A multi perspective study

Südwestdeutscher Verlag für Hochschulschriften

**Impressum/Imprint (nur für Deutschland/only for Germany)**
Bibliografische Information der Deutschen Nationalbibliothek: Die Deutsche Nationalbibliothek verzeichnet diese Publikation in der Deutschen Nationalbibliografie; detaillierte bibliografische Daten sind im Internet über http://dnb.d-nb.de abrufbar.
Alle in diesem Buch genannten Marken und Produktnamen unterliegen warenzeichen-, marken- oder patentrechtlichem Schutz bzw. sind Warenzeichen oder eingetragene Warenzeichen der jeweiligen Inhaber. Die Wiedergabe von Marken, Produktnamen, Gebrauchsnamen, Handelsnamen, Warenbezeichnungen u.s.w. in diesem Werk berechtigt auch ohne besondere Kennzeichnung nicht zu der Annahme, dass solche Namen im Sinne der Warenzeichen- und Markenschutzgesetzgebung als frei zu betrachten wären und daher von jedermann benutzt werden dürften.

Coverbild: www.ingimage.com

Verlag: Südwestdeutscher Verlag für Hochschulschriften GmbH & Co. KG
Heinrich-Böcking-Str. 6-8, 66121 Saarbrücken, Deutschland
Telefon +49 681 37 20 271-1, Telefax +49 681 37 20 271-0
Email: info@svh-verlag.de

Approved by: Zürich, ETH, Diss., 2009

Herstellung in Deutschland:
Schaltungsdienst Lange o.H.G., Berlin
Books on Demand GmbH, Norderstedt
Reha GmbH, Saarbrücken
Amazon Distribution GmbH, Leipzig
**ISBN: 978-3-8381-2968-6**

**Imprint (only for USA, GB)**
Bibliographic information published by the Deutsche Nationalbibliothek: The Deutsche Nationalbibliothek lists this publication in the Deutsche Nationalbibliografie; detailed bibliographic data are available in the Internet at http://dnb.d-nb.de.
Any brand names and product names mentioned in this book are subject to trademark, brand or patent protection and are trademarks or registered trademarks of their respective holders. The use of brand names, product names, common names, trade names, product descriptions etc. even without a particular marking in this works is in no way to be construed to mean that such names may be regarded as unrestricted in respect of trademark and brand protection legislation and could thus be used by anyone.

Cover image: www.ingimage.com

Publisher: Südwestdeutscher Verlag für Hochschulschriften GmbH & Co. KG
Heinrich-Böcking-Str. 6-8, 66121 Saarbrücken, Germany
Phone +49 681 37 20 271-1, Fax +49 681 37 20 271-0
Email: info@svh-verlag.de

Printed in the U.S.A.
Printed in the U.K. by (see last page)
**ISBN: 978-3-8381-2968-6**

Copyright © 2012 by the author and Südwestdeutscher Verlag für Hochschulschriften GmbH & Co. KG and licensors
All rights reserved. Saarbrücken 2012

# Contents

Abstract .................................................................................................................. I
List of abbreviations ............................................................................................. III

## 1 INTRODUCTION AND OUTLINE ............................................................... 1
  1.1 Introduction .................................................................................................. 1
  1.2 Objectives of the thesis ................................................................................ 2
  1.3 Outline of the thesis ..................................................................................... 3

## 2 BACKGROUND ............................................................................................. 5
  2.1 Emotion ........................................................................................................ 5
    2.1.1 *A short foreword to emotion research* ................................................. 6
    2.1.2 *The emotional brain* ............................................................................ 7
    2.1.3 *What is an emotion?* ........................................................................... 8
    2.1.4 *On the relationship between emotion, cognition and behaviour* ........ 9
  2.2 Pain ............................................................................................................. 10
    2.2.1 *Nociceptive pathways and brain regions* .......................................... 12
    2.2.2 *Top-Down modulation of pain* .......................................................... 13
    2.2.3 *The endogenous opioid system* ......................................................... 13
  2.3 Emotional and cognitive modulations of pain ............................................ 15
    2.3.1 *Attention, anticipation and expectation of pain relief* ...................... 16
    2.3.2 *Perceived control* .............................................................................. 17
    2.3.3 *Reappraisal and perceived self-identity* ........................................... 18
    2.3.4 *Positive and negative emotions* ........................................................ 19
    2.3.5 *Endogenous opioids and the regulation of pain and emotion* .......... 20

## 3 MATERIALS AND METHODS ................................................................... 23
  3.1 Subjects ...................................................................................................... 23
  3.2 Pain stimuli ................................................................................................. 23
  3.3 Emotional stimuli ....................................................................................... 24
    3.3.1 *Role induction* ................................................................................... 24
    3.3.2 *Pleasure induction* ............................................................................ 25
  3.4 Autonomic reactivity .................................................................................. 26
    3.4.1 *Skin conductance level* ..................................................................... 26
    3.4.2 *Startle eyeblink response* .................................................................. 27
    3.4.3 *Voice measurement* ........................................................................... 28
  3.5 Subjective reports ....................................................................................... 28
    3.5.1 *Subjective ratings of pain* ................................................................. 28
    3.5.2 *Subjective ratings of emotions and mood* ........................................ 29
    3.5.3 *Subjective ratings of role empathy and meaningfulness* .................. 29
  3.6 Statistical analysis ...................................................................................... 30
  3.7 Medication .................................................................................................. 30
    3.7.1 *Pharmacodynamic und pharmacokinetic properties of naloxone* .... 30

# 4 PSYCHOPHYSICS OF PAIN ........................................................... 33

- 4.1 Objectives and hypotheses of the study ................................................ 33
- 4.2 Design and methods of the study ......................................................... 34
  - 4.2.1 Data analysis ............................................................................... 35
- 4.3 Results ..................................................................................................... 35
  - 4.3.1 Pain threshold ............................................................................. 35
  - 4.3.2 Pain tolerance ............................................................................. 36
- 4.4 Discussion ............................................................................................... 38
- 4.5 Conclusion .............................................................................................. 42

# 5 ROLE-IDENTITY AND PAIN ...................................................... 43

- 5.1 Objectives and hypotheses of the study ................................................ 45
- 5.2 Design and methods of the study ......................................................... 45
  - 5.2.1 Data analysis ............................................................................... 47
- 5.3 Results ..................................................................................................... 48
  - 5.3.1 Pain tolerance and threshold ..................................................... 48
  - 5.3.2 McGill pain questionnaire (MPQ) .............................................. 49
  - 5.3.3 Visual analogue scale (VAS) for pain intensity and unpleasantness ......... 51
  - 5.3.4 Role-play questionnaire ............................................................. 51
  - 5.3.5 Autonomic responses ................................................................. 52
  - 5.3.6 Voice measurement .................................................................... 53
- 5.4 Discussion ............................................................................................... 53
- 5.5 Conclusion .............................................................................................. 57

# 6 NEUROCHEMISTRY OF PLEASURE-RELATED ANALGESIA ............... 59

- 6.1 Objectives and hypotheses of the study ................................................ 59
- 6.2 Design and methods of the study ......................................................... 60
  - 6.2.1 Data analysis ............................................................................... 62
- 6.3 Results ..................................................................................................... 62
  - 6.3.1 Expectation ................................................................................. 62
  - 6.3.2 Pain tolerance ............................................................................. 63
  - 6.3.3 Subjective ratings of pain .......................................................... 64
  - 6.3.4 Subjective ratings of emotion ................................................... 64
  - 6.3.5 Autonomic responses ................................................................. 65
  - 6.3.6 Mood ............................................................................................ 66
- 6.4 Discussion ............................................................................................... 66
- 6.5 Conclusion .............................................................................................. 68

# 7 SYNTHESIS AND OUTLOOK ...................................................... 71

- 7.1 Synthesis ................................................................................................. 71
- I. .................................................................................................................... 71
  - The hurtfulness of pain ................................................................... 71
  - Homeostasis ..................................................................................... 72
  - "I am in pain" ................................................................................... 73
  - On self-images ................................................................................. 74
  - Meeting the role expectations ....................................................... 75
  - The status of employment as a substantive part of self-esteem ......... 76
  - Feelings of control .......................................................................... 77
  - The willingness to endure pain ..................................................... 78

|       | What neural circuits are involved? | 79 |
|---|---|---|
| II.   |                                    | 80 |
|       | The endeavour to design a follow-up study | 80 |
|       | Pain and pleasure | 81 |
|       | Pleasure-related analgesia | 82 |
|       | Pain: imprinting and being imprinted | 83 |
|       | Activation of opioid circuits | 84 |
|       | Placebo, naloxone and the pain-modulatory system | 85 |
|       | Naloxone-sensitive and –insensitive inhibitory pathways | 86 |
|       | Non-opioid mechanisms | 86 |
|       | Receptor affinities and pharmacological antagonisation | 88 |
|       | Women and men | 90 |
| III.  |                                    | 91 |
|       | "Reflection kills desire" | 91 |
|       | Emotion induction | 92 |
|       | Pleasure in the brain | 94 |
|       | Mind as real as matter? | 95 |
|       | Molecular feelings | 96 |
| 7.2   | SUMMARY AND CONCLUSION | 97 |
| 7.3   | OUTLOOK | 99 |

# 8 APPENDIX ... 101

| 8.1 | REFERENCES | 101 |
|---|---|---|

# Abstract

Emotions are a whole-body event. They encompass arousal, bodily expression, action tendencies, attentional orientation, and affective feeling, and have been recognized to be of global importance for human experience and behaviour. When we are cheerful, heart-broken, nervous or furious we may for example decide, speak, taste and concentrate differently and become selective in what we recall. The experiential consequences and neurobiological mechanisms underlying emotional modulation of perception can be extensively studied in pain. The notion of pain as a purely sensory experience has given way to a multi-dimensional view. Pain is not a simple 1:1 response to a nociceptive stimulus, but is influenced by pathological and genetic factors, and is further subject to a complex set of individual, contextual, and environmental variables. These factors are regulated by diverse modulatory circuits within the central nervous system and have gained increased interest in pain research.

Within the scope of this thesis three studies were conducted that investigated emotional modulation of experimental heat pain in healthy volunteers, focusing both on the experiential level and underlying neurochemical mechanisms. The first methodological study (*psychophysics study*) demonstrated that experimental heat pain delivered to the volar forearm does not differ in pain threshold and tolerance measurements within and across forearm sites. It is therefore a suitable way to investigate individual pain perception in experimental and clinical settings.

In the second study (*role-identity study*) the focus was turned to contextual and emotional aspects of pain perception. The induction of two opposing roles, a *hero/heroine* and *faint-heart*, reshaped the attribution of meaningfulness and the will to endure pain, further the emotional state, which in the end affected intensity and quality of pain perception.

The third study (*opioid study*) approached the neurochemical underpinnings of emotional pain modulation. Since endogenous opioids have often been associated with the regulation of both pain and emotion, it was hypothesized that enhanced μ-opioidergic neurotransmission during positive emotional states leads to diminished pain perception. However, despite complete μ-opioid receptor blockade with naloxone pleasure-related increases in pain tolerance were not affected, while subjective pain ratings increased. Strikingly, these results revealed that besides μ-opioid neurotransmission, non-opioid mediated circuits play a major role in the emotional modulation of pain perception.

The findings of this thesis clearly demonstrate that pain is a dynamic experience, by which noxious stimuli are permanently modulated and re-evaluated within a broader context of the individual and its interaction with the environment. Emotional states are thereby associated with an intricate interplay of co-ordinated neurotransmitter systems that lead to endogenous pain modulation. The acknowledgment of the organism as a unity, where mental phenomena cannot be separated from their physical consequences, shapes our understanding of 'bodily' and 'emotional' homeostasis. It should therefore be of great value for both the pharmacological care of pain patients and also the individual and clinical management of other challenges in life.

—

Every research endeavour is shaped by its scientific environment. The present work was developed from 2004–2009 at the transdisciplinary institute Collegium Helveticum of the University of Zurich and Swiss Federal Institute of Technology Zurich (ETH Dissertation No 18604). It is part of the research project: "The role of emotion: Its part in human behaviour and setting of social norms". At the Collegium Helveticum, I had the opportunity and the privilege to discuss the topic from different perspectives with peers from other scientific disciplines, which helped me to sharpen and refine my research questions and interpret the findings. I will treasure my time as a PhD student at the institute and I am grateful for the support and companionship of many people that have helped me in doing my research, and in the mean time have provided me with *social joy*.

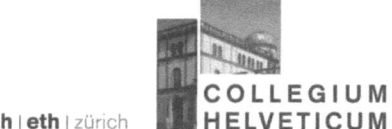

# List of abbreviations

| | |
|---|---|
| ANOVA | Analysis of variance |
| EEG | Electroencephalography |
| EMG | Electromyography |
| ETH | Swiss Federal Institute of Technology Zurich |
| fMRI | Functional magnetic resonance imaging |
| IAPS | International affective picture system |
| i.v. | Intravenous administration |
| $K_i$ | Dissociation constant |
| MDBF | Mehrdimensionaler Befindlichkeitsfragebogen |
| MEG | Magnetoencephalography |
| MPQ | McGill pain questionnaire |
| NaCl | Sodium chloride |
| PET | Positron emission tomography |
| p | Significance level |
| SAM | Self-assessment manikin (questionnaire) |
| SCL | Skin conductance level |
| S.D. | Standard deviation |
| S.E. | Standard error |
| s.c. | Subcutaneous application |
| UZH | University of Zurich |
| VAS | Visual analogue scale |

# 1
# Introduction and Outline

At the start of the 21st century, neuroscience has developed into a genuinely interdisciplinary field, uniting a wide variety of disciplinary expertise in medicine, biology, chemistry, pharmacology, psychology, engineering, mathematics, philosophy and many more. Like the field of genetics, neuroscience concerns the biological foundations of who we are, and how we work. Particularly, the research on emotion[1] has changed from being a field fraught with too many difficulties to be considered as a tractable topic of study, to a 'hot topic'. This growing interest in the neurobiology of emotion parallels a wider recognition of its global importance to human experience and behaviour. Pain is a substantial and thoroughly subjective sensory experience that is modulated by emotion. As a fundamental constant of life, it prevails at the moment of birth – and oftentimes at the moment of death. Fascinatingly, pain, which is the sensation that arises from a nociceptive input, is not only influenced by 'physiological' factors, such as pathological or genetic condition, but also by 'psychological' factors, such as beliefs, prior experiences, attitudes and emotions. It is therefore an insightful field for the study of how emotions affect human experiences.

## 1.1    Introduction

The idea that sensory experience is shaped by one's attitudes, beliefs and emotions, has gained currency among psychologists, physicians, and the general public (Wager et al., 2004). In this line of reasoning, pain is seen as a dynamic multidimensional experience entailing not only *sensory-discriminative* components, but also *cognitive-*

---

[1] What emotions are and whether they differ from feelings is elaborated in chap. 2.1.3.

*evaluative*, and *affective-motivational* dimensions (Melzack and Casey, 1968).[2] It has been recognized that noxious stimuli originating from actual or potential tissue damage are evaluated and modulated in higher brain areas, encompassing cognitive, emotional, and motivational dimensions.

Pain has a vital function in life. As an 'alarm system' it sustains homeostasis, by increasing avoidance from a threat to the organism, or guiding attention to an injured or malfunctioning body part. However, pain can loose its meaning, become intractable and develop into a chronic state, as seen for example in phantom limb or neuropathic pain. In this case, pain is no longer considered a symptom but an illness by itself. Chronic pain has major negative effects on millions of patients worldwide, and causes tremendous costs for the health care system. The vast majority of research on pain control has concentrated on peripheral and spinal cord mechanisms of opioid and anti-inflammatory analgesic therapy and breakthroughs have been rare in the past fifty years (Melzack, 2008). Now, western medicine is increasingly giving credence to a patient's own ability to modify pain. The research on the widely known placebo effect, for example, has provided evidence that cognitive processes connected to the expectation of treatment and recovery are associated with the mobilization of internal mechanisms, eliciting an objectively observable physiological response (Zubieta and Stohler, 2009). Unravelling emotional and cognitive modulation of pain and the underlying neuroanatomical and neurochemical factors that contribute to endogenous pain inhibition has become an essential element in the study and treatment of pain (Magnusson and Fisher, 2000).

## 1.2  Objectives of the thesis

This thesis is embedded in the transdisciplinary research project of the Collegium Helveticum during the years 2004–2009 on emotion entitled "Die Rolle der Emotion: ihr Anteil bei menschlichem Handeln und bei der Setzung sozialer Normen" (The role of emotion: Its part in human behaviour and setting of social norms). The overall objective of the thesis was to investigate different aspects of emotional modulation of pain perception. The first aim was, to set a methodological basis for experimental heat pain measurements: an experimental study analyzed, whether different sites on

---

[2] The three dimensions of pain can be described with various adjectives, as for instance pricking, cramping, crushing, and wrenching for the *sensory-discriminative* dimension, annoying, miserable, unbearable for the *cognitive-evaluative* dimension, and tiring, sickening, terrifying, cruel for the *affective-motivational* dimension (Melzack, 1975).

the forearms of healthy study participants show side symmetries in pain threshold and tolerance measurements. Then, previous findings, showing that positive emotions lead to a decrease of pain perception, while negative emotions to an increase, were analyzed in a broader context. A study in healthy volunteers investigated the effects of self-perceived role identity and concomitant emotions on pain perception, including such aspects as meaningfulness, and gender differences. A third clinical study addressed the neurochemistry underlying the analgesic effects of positive emotional states on pain. The aim was to verify, whether endogenous opioids mediate pleasure-related analgesia and can thus be regarded as 'molecular interfaces' between pain and emotions.

## 1.3  Outline of the thesis

The thesis is based on the findings of three experimental studies in healthy volunteers investigating emotional modulation of pain perception.

Chapter 2 gives an overview on emotion and pain research. More specifically, it gives insight into the history of emotion research and outlines current knowledge on the neurobiological bases of emotion. Moreover, the neural pathways of pain processing are described and an overview on recent findings on emotional and cognitive modulation of pain perception is given.

Chapter 3 describes materials and methods that were used in the three experimental studies. Furthermore, details on statistical analyses can be found here.

Chapter 4 presents the findings of the methodological study on the psychophysics of experimental heat pain measurements (*psychophysics study*). The characterization of pain threshold and tolerances of the human forearm in healthy volunteers provides a solid basis for experimental or clinical setting where pain measurements are the parameter of interest.

Chapter 5 reports the findings on self-perceived role identity on pain (*role-identity study*). It shows that perceiving oneself as a *hero/heroine* versus a *faint-heart* in a painful context changes emotional state and meaningfulness of noxious stimuli and leads to altered pain tolerance and pain unpleasantness.

Chapter 6 illustrates the experiments on the role of endogenous opioid neurotransmission in emotional modulation of pain (*opioid study*). Pharmacological blockade of the neurotransmitter system indicates that besides opioid- mainly non-opioid mediated nociceptive circuits contribute to pleasure-related analgesia.

In chapter 7 the paradigms and results of the experimental studies are joined in an overall discussion and synthesis. Particularly, different ideas, concepts, and views that accompanied my thesis at the Collegium Helveticum and that are beyond the scope of disciplinary scientific publication can be found here. A summary, conclusion and outlook on future pain research close this chapter.

# 2
# Background

Etymology tells us that the word 'emotion' (from the Latin verb emovere) literally means an outward movement. Emotion is the welling up of an impulse within that tends towards outward expression and action. For centuries the study of this "welling up" has been in the realm of philosophers, as for example Aristotle, Descartes, Spinoza, Hume and Kant (Demmerling and Landweer, 2007). In the last 130 years (see below) psychology and disciplines from the field of natural sciences have found increased interest in the understanding of the neurobiology of emotions. Nowadays, miscellaneous theoretical frameworks accounting for the diverse aspects of emotion – from the biological to psychological to phenomenological – can be found. Many of them try to elucidate the impact of emotion on human perception and behaviour in conceptually and empirically profitable ways. The role of emotion in the perception and modulation of *pain* is the focus of this thesis. In the following an outline on recent findings from the field of neuroscience on emotions, pain and their interactions will be given.

## 2.1  Emotion

What were we without emotions? They are the colour, the spice, the treasure, and scourge, in short, the engine of our lives. Every experience is shaped by emotion, influencing its quality and range. Emotions index occurrences of value to events in the world, be it in physical or sociocultural contexts, or most evidently in human and animal relationships. In terms of homeostasis emotions are a motivation system that either rewards or punishes our behaviour. Emotions can be bliss, equally misery and heartbreak and are a good many times ambivalent. Even though the notion is ubiquitous these days in human- and natural sciences and media, different individuals – laymen and scientists alike – struggle and disagree in answering the straightforward question: what is an emotion?

### 2.1.1 A short foreword to emotion research

Of course, William James. It was his essay *"What is an emotion"* that pioneered the psychological and neurobiological science of emotions in 1884 (James, 1884). James postulated that emotions are the result of the experience of sets of bodily changes that occur in response to emotional stimuli. We are sad because we cry, and not the other way around. Since Carl Lange provided similar ideas at around the same time (1885) the theory that emotional reactions in the body must precede a feeling of emotion is known as the James-Lange theory of emotions.

Already, in 1872 Charles Darwin had published his groundbreaking book *"The expression of the emotions in man and animals"* where he proposed that a distinct set of fundamental emotions such as anger, fear, surprise, sadness, are homologous across species and cultures (Darwin, 1872/1998). Darwin's observations gave rise to the use of animals in research to understand emotions in humans. In the 1920'ies Walter B. Cannon and Philip Bard who used cats as animal lesion models challenged the James-Lange theory. On the logic that changes in behaviour after surgery reflect processes that involve the lesioned part of the brain, they were able to show that anger response also exists after removal of parts of the sensory and motor cortices. Furthermore, the total surgical separation of the viscera from the brain did not impair emotional behaviour, indicating that the viscera and innervation of muscles are not the sources for the qualities of emotion (Cannon, 1927).

Most interestingly, this debate is still continuing and finds renewed vigor by publications of Ekman (Ekman and Davidson, 1994) and Niedenthal (Niedenthal, 2007) on embodied emotions. These contemporary neuroscientists re-establish a modified James-Lange view by giving evidence that bodily reactions, such as mimic or posture, causally affect how emotional information is processed. In 1937 James Papez introduced the concept of a central neural circuitry of emotions and was the first in postulating a neural network theory for emotions (Papez, 1937). Another fifteen years later Paul MacLean came up with a sound concept that has survived to the current day, although by now somewhat outdated (Calder et al., 2001; Pessoa, 2008). It is the notion of a 'limbic system' as the localy defined 'seat of emotions' (Maclean, 1952).

For the next thirty years neuroscientific emotion research came to a halt. This might have been in part due to the emergence of cognitive science, as a reaction to the dominance of behaviourism at the time (Miller, 2003). The cognitive revolution based on a computer metaphor of the brain and left no room for emotion. Researchers embraced cognitive questions free from fuzzy and hardly tractable subjective emotional experiences. By doing so, they were also released from having to solve the mind-body problem (LeDoux, 2000).[3] Since the 1980ies we have witnessed an "explosion in affective neuroscience" (Dalgleish, 2004). Over these years, the 'emotional brain', i.e. the set of regions that processes emotions, has fluctuated considerably. Nevertheless, some regions have consistently been linked to emotional processes, although none can be ascribed as "purely affective" (Pessoa, 2008).

## 2.1.2 The emotional brain

Drawing a map of the set of brain regions that constitute the emotional brain is "plagued by possibly insurmountable conceptual difficulties" (Pessoa, 2008). Up to this day, an impressive body of neuroscientific literature is trying to understand what emotion is from neurobiological perspective. As elaborated before, neuroscientists have come to the general agreement that emotions are embodied in the brain, although of course, other scholars would argue on this biologistic notion. The central question posed by affective neuroscience is: *how* are emotions encoded in the brain. Which brain circuits underlie emotions and are there different neural systems for different emotions? Diverse methods have been developed and are being used such as, animal and human behavioural experiments and lesion studies, electrophysiological recordings, and functional neuroimaging. However, the plethora of literature pinpointing regions where emotional information enters, travels through and exits, might not be conclusive. Most intriguingly, the question has come up whether emotion is rather an emergent property of the whole brain neural network then the interaction of a limited set of regions (Blanchard et al., 2001). A very interesting field of research carefully considers the brain connectivities, since "a given brain region is only a few synapses away from every other brain region" (Pessoa, 2008). Recent developments in the quantitative analysis of complex networks in network science suggest that the brain has a 'small-world' architecture (Bullmore and Sporns, 2009). A 'small-world' property means that nodes of a network are highly clustered, for instance cortical areas, and short paths globally link all nodes of the network through relatively few intermediate steps.[4] For example, the amygdala, since 1937 one of the most thorough investigated regions in the neural system of emotion (Phelps, 2006), occupies a posi-

---

[3] How current research rejoins emotion and cognition will be discussed in chap. 2.1.4.
[4] On a sidenote, the connectivity graphs of the interactions at the Collegium Helveticum (Ulbrich, 2011) nicely resemble the small world topology of brain connectivity graphs as for example depicted in Pessoa, 2008, p. 152.

tion at the very geometric centre of the topological map of the brain network (Swanson, 2003). Network studies on structural and temporal connectivity emphasize that brain areas do not work in isolation, but instead are part of intersecting networks with which they are affiliated at a particular time.

### 2.1.3 What is an emotion?

> "Defining 'emotion' is a notorious problem."
> – Klaus R. Scherer, 2005

The proceeding sections addressed the neurobiological fundamentals of how emotions are encoded in the brain leaving out the psychophysical dimensions and their substantial bodily consequences. Klaus R. Scherer, a renowned emotion researcher in Geneva, concludes that "the number of scientific definitions proposed has grown to the point where counting seems quite hopeless" (Scherer 05). However, when searching for a definition in a scientific paper, review, or handbook, as for instance in the "*Handbook of Emotions*" (Lewis and Haviland-Jones, 2000) or "*Handbook of Affective Sciences*" (Davidson et al., 2003)) one comes to realize that authors most often simply avoid raising this question. Obviously, the abundance of emotion definitions arises from the broad philosophical and scientific frameworks and methodologies involved in the conceptualization of emotion. Within the scope of the present work I would like to cite two approaches subsuming emotion.

Evan Thompson, who worked closely with the biologist and philosopher Francisco Varela, describes emotion in his new book "*Mind in Life*" (Thompson, 2007) as follows: "(…) emotion is a prototype whole-organism event, for it mobilizes and coordinates virtually every aspect of the organism. Emotion involves the entire neuraxis of brain stem, limbic areas, and superior cortex, as well as visceral and motor processes of the body. It encompasses psychosomatic networks of molecular communication among the nervous system, immune system, and endocrine system." Another prevailing view of emotion has been put forward by Antonio Damasio. He uses the term emotion to designate a collection of responses triggered from parts of the brain to the body, and within the brain, using both neural and neurochemical pathways ((Damasio, 1994; Damasio, 1998). The end result of the collection of such neural, humoral, visceral and musco-skeletal responses, such as alterations in hormone level, heart rate, skin conductance and muscle tension, in the whole organism is an *emotional state*. In contrast, the term *feeling* describes the complex mental state that results from the emotional state.

## 2.1.4 On the relationship between emotion, cognition and behaviour

> "In jedem Gefühl sind Denkakte, Bewertungs-
> und Abstraktionsakte vorhanden."
> – Michael von Brück, 2006

The dichotomy between emotion and cognition has a very long tradition in Western philosophy. The rationalist view that rational thinking precedes emotion in the ways of acquiring knowledge has strongly influenced our conception of the mind. In the last century the superiority of cognition over emotion was additionally emphasized by the notion that emotions are somehow limbic and subcortical and cognition cortical and thus higher order (Maclean, 1952). Moreover, the computer metaphor, coined during the cognitive revolution, helped propagate the sterile approach to the mind as an information-processing device free of blurring emotion. But how could it possibly be that cognition, including perception, attention, evaluation, memory, planning, reflection, and decision making, is free from emotion? In everyday life behaviour and experience cognitive processes are seamlessly integrated with emotions including arousal, action tendencies, bodily expression, attentional orientation, and affective feeling, though certainly to a greater or lesser extent depending on the context. Emotions can shape virtually all aspects of cognition. When we are cheerful, heart-broken, nervous or furious we may for example decide, drive, concentrate, and recall differently. The evaluation of a situation's significance, it's appraisal, thus is rather an emergent global state of the mind that constitutes of cognitive and emotional networks (Thompson, 2007). In fact, studies on the neural substrates of emotional and cognitive processes evidence no clear segregation (Dolan, 2002; LeDoux, 2000). Moreover, there is a large amount of anatomical overlap between the neural systems mediating cognition and emotion processes, and these systems interact with each other in a reciprocal and circular way (Pessoa, 2008). Eventually, the complementarity of emotion and cognition also finds resonance in current philosophical and neuroscientific approaches towards a cognitive or rational significance of emotion (Damasio, 1994; Gladwell, 2005).

An emerging and increasingly popular theme in neuroscience is the question of *how* emotions interact with processes, such as attention, memory, learning, reasoning, and decision-making (Davidson et al., 2003; Lewis and Haviland-Jones, 2000). But one can start to investigate emotional interactions even one step ahead: at the level of perception of external and internal inputs. First, how do we perceive for example visual, auditory, or sensual stimuli dependent on their emotional quality, and second, do they evoke appropriate responses such as feelings, judgments and behaviour? The experiential consequences and the mechanisms underlying the emotional modulation of perception can be extensively studied in pain perception. This research field thereby transcends the classical categories of 'physiological' and 'psychological dimensions of human experience that are based on a dualistic view of the mind-body problem and have a long tradition in Western philosophy (Goldie, 2000; Stich and Warfield, 2002).

## 2.2 Pain

Pain is a highly unpleasant sensation. Once triggered it can act as a potent motivational drive and thoroughly dominate attention. The International Association for the Study of Pain defines pain, as "an unpleasant *sensory and emotional* experience associated with *actual or potential* tissue damage, or described in terms of such damage" (Merskey and Bogduk, 1994). This wide definition of pain recognizes that the subjective experience of pain is modulated by a complex set of individual, contextual, and environmental variables. Pain, which is the interpretation of a nociceptive input, is not only influenced by pathological and genetic factors, but is also subject to memories, beliefs, expectations, attitudes, and emotions. Thus, the resultant percept is not necessarily related linearly to the nociceptive drive or input. The definition emphasizes another characteristic of pain: its Janus-like duality. Pain serves simultaneously as a discriminative sensation and as a global sign of danger to the physical or psychological equilibrium. Unfortunately, pain sometimes detaches from its vital protective function. This is especially true when pain persists for more than three months, which is then called a chronic pain state. Chronic pain has become one of the largest medical health problems in the developed world. According to a European pain survey chronic pain of moderate to severe intensity occurs in 19% of adult Europeans, seriously affecting the quality of their social and working lives. Very few are managed by pain specialists and nearly half receive inadequate pain management (Breivik et al., 2006). A recent study estimated total health care expenditures incurred by individuals with back pain in the United States of 90.7 billion US dollars, which represented at the time 1 percent of the U.S. Gross Domestic Product (Luo et al., 2004).

The highly subjective nature of pain makes it difficult to assess. There is no approach to pain without acknowledging that there is a difference between the *first person* perspective, of the individual who is in pain, and the *third person* perspective of the doctor or experimenter who is trying to measure the pain.[5] An experimenter can objectively determine pain tolerance of a study participant, by measuring for example the time the participant bears to hold his or her hand in icy water, or sustains heat on the skin. But the observer will have insurmountable problems to determine the subjective dimension of pain the participant experiences at that moment (see chap. 7). Solely by measuring objective parameters from the outside one cannot know *how* the pain of a participant or patient *feels like*. Thomas Nagel depicted the phenomenon that the nature of subjective experience can never be known by objective knowledge from the outside in his famous paper "*What is it like to be a bat?*" (Nagel, 1974). Nevertheless, researchers and care-givers are in constant effort to tackle the first person perspective of pain as adequately as possible. As in most experimental pain studies, the experiments in this thesis assessed both the objective and subjective dimensions of pain.[6] Strikingly, the *opioid study* demonstrated how the two dimensions can diverge and show differing results upon neurotransmitter blockade (see chap. 6 ).

As Apkarian et al. put it, "up to twenty years ago, our understanding of the role of the brain, above the spinal cord, in pain processing was limited and based primarily on animal anatomical and electrophysiological studies" (Apkarian et al., 2005). The advent of non-invasive brain imaging techniques, allowing for comparisons between conscious healthy subjects and clinical pain patients, has lead to a veritable revolution of concepts. In the pain field, there is now growing recognition that a variety of pain modulatory mechanisms exist in the nervous system, and these modulatory systems can be accessed either pharmacologically or through contextual and/or mental manipulation. More and more, studies addressing possible neural mechanisms underlying each of these influences are being developed and reveal astonishing insights into how the brain functions at the interface of 'mind' and 'body' (Ingvar, 1999; Rainville, 2002; Tracey and Mantyh, 2007; Wiech et al., 2008b). In the following sections an introduction to today's understanding of nociceptive processing in the central nervous system and emerging evidence on mental pain modulatory systems shall be given.

---

[5] For more discussion on the observer problem in the assessment of pain and emotion please refer to (Folkers and Wittwer, 2007).
[6] Pain perception was determined by measuring heat pain threshold and tolerance (in °C) and subjective ratings of pain intensity and unpleasantness using visual analogue scales and a choice of pain describing adjectives (see chap. 3 ).

## 2.2.1 Nociceptive pathways and brain regions

Physical pain usually stems from potentially damaging environmental stimuli such as extreme temperature, pressure, distention, noxious chemicals, or tissue damage that activate nociceptors in the tissues. From there, actions potentials are transmitted to neurons in the dorsal horn of the spinal cord through fast A-delta fibers (approx. 20m/sec) and slower C fibers (approx. 2m/sec). Further processing in the dorsal roots, trigeminal nuclei and spinal cord can involve intricate circuits of opioid, cannabinoid and NMDA (N-Methyl-D-Aspartat) receptors, specific protein kinases, and further modulation by substances such as substances P and K, serotonin, extracellular protons, arachidonic acid, bradykinin, nucleotides, calcitonin gene-related peptide, and neurotrophins (Ribeiro et al., 2005). From the dorsal horn cells, ascending spinal pathways project into multiple brain areas (Price, 2000). Several brain areas have been specified to play a role in pain processing, but are not unequivocally defined (Tracey and Mantyh, 2007). Studies using positron emission tomography (PET), functional magnetic resonance imaging (fMRI), electroencephalography (EEG), and magnetoencephalography (MEG) have mainly found activity in the following brain areas during acute pain: primary and secondary somatosensory, insular, anterior cingulated, and prefontal cortices as well as the thalamus (Apkarian et al., 2005). Depending on the set of contextual and individual variables, such as the type of pain stimulus and influences of the overall status of the body, also regions as the basal ganglia, cerebellum, amygdala, hippocampus, and areas within the parietal and temporal cortices can be involved (Tracey and Mantyh, 2007).

Most interestingly, nociceptive information is processed both 'in series' and 'in parallel'. Ascending spinal pathways project (1) directly into brainstem and limbic areas, where nociceptive information is integrated with essential homeostatic, arousal and autonomic processes, and (2) indirectly from somatosensory cortical areas to cortical limbic structures, where it is cognitively mediated (Price, 2000). Both ascending nociceptive pathways – the direct and the cortico-limbic pathway – converge on the same anterior cingulated cortical and subcortical structures. The function of these key areas may be to interrelate attentional and evaluative functions with emotional valence. Via further cognitive projection and evaluation in the prefrontal cortex also response priorities can be assigned (Price, 2002).

## 2.2.2 Top-Down modulation of pain

As described above, pain is by its very nature a multifactorial and highly subjective experience. It is not a simple 1:1 response to a nociceptive stimulus, but is regulated by diverse modulatory circuits within the central nervous system. In addition to the ascending nociceptive pathways, recent findings describe putative descending modulatory pathways (Millan, 2002). These dynamic 'top-down' (neural effects from higher to lower brain levels) processes are able to amplify, attenuate, shape, or color the pain experience. Having modulatory power they are thought to play a crucial role in adaptive and maladaptive reactions to pain. They originate in cerebral cortical areas including the amygdala and project through hypothalamic and brainstem structures to the dorsal horn where both inhibitory (antinociceptive) and facilitatory (pronociceptive) effects are exerted. It is thus interesting to note, that pain can be bi-directionally regulated at the level of the dorsal horn (Fields, 2004; Price, 2002). Knowledge on the anatomical network of these descending pain modulatory systems largely came from animal studies, where it was shown that electrical stimulation of the brainstem can produce analgesia (Basbaum and Fields, 1984). Later work postulated that main parts of these systems are sensitive to opioids and contribute to opioid analgesia induced by both exogenous or endogenous origin (Fields, 2004).

## 2.2.3 The endogenous opioid system

The endogenous opioid system, termed colloquially as the 'heroin within', has fascinated researchers and the public for the last 40 years. It consists of several G-protein coupled receptors with multiple subtypes, named μ (mu, for morphine, named after Morpheus, the Greek god of dreams), κ (kappa), δ (delta), ORL1 (for opioid receptor-like) that were discovered and described since the beginning of the 1970ies.[7] Opioid receptors are distributed throughout the central nervous system and peripheral tissue, whereby localization and functions of the subtypes differ. They are regulated by receptor desensitization, internalization, resensitization, and downregulation (Raehal and Bohn, 2005). The endogenous neuropeptides belong to different families: endorphins, enkephalins, dynorphins, nociceptins, and recently discovered endomorphins (Zadina et al., 1997). Neurones producing these neuropeptides can be identified using messenger RNA probes for their precursor proteines (Dickenson, 1997). The precursor proteins are pre-pro-opiomelanocortin, pre-pro-enkephalin, pre-pro-dynorphin,

---

[7] For a detailed list of first publications please consult Ribeiro et al., 2005, p. 1267.

pre-pro-endomorphin (Table 1). Studies on mice with targeted disruptions of opioid-receptor and peptide genes have lead to important insights into the function of the endogenous opioid system suggesting its involvement in the regulation of pain, and furthermore emotion, autonomic, and endocrine function (Bodnar, 2008; McNally and Akil, 2002).

Table 1: **Summary of the various families of opioid peptides and their receptors.** The list is derived from (Millan, 2002) and not exhaustive. ENK = enkephalin, DYN = dynorphin; POMC = pro-opiomelanocortin, β-EP = β-endorphin, DH = dorsal horn, PAG = periaqueductal grey, RVM = rostroventral medulla.

| Precursor | Product(s) | Receptor(s) | Site(s) of action |
|---|---|---|---|
| Pre-pro-ENK | Met- and Leu-ENK | δ | DH, PAG, amygdala, RVM |
| Pre-pro-DYN | DYN | κ | DH, PAG, amygdala, RVM |
| Pre-pro-endomorphin | Endomorphin 1 and 2 | μ | DH, PAG, amygdala |
| | Endomorphin 1 and 2 | δ/κ | DH (via ENK/DYN) |
| Pre-POMC | β-EP | μ | DH, amygdala, PAG |

There is consensus that the analgesic effects of opioids arise from their ability to inhibit directly the ascending transmission of nociceptive information, and from their ability to activate descending pain control circuits (Fields, 2004; McNally and Akil, 2002). Pain studies have focused largely on the μ-opioid receptor, because its activation is necessary for the analgesic action of endogenous and exogenous opioids, such as morphine. Novel in-vivo brain imaging techniques allow for determination of distribution and stimulus-related activation of opioid receptors in the conscious human. In these ligand-PET pain studies, mainly the selective μ-opioid agonist radiotracer [$^{11}$C]carfentanil and the unspecific opioid receptor antagonist [$^{11}$C]diprenorphine are used (Sprenger et al., 2005). Activation of the endogenous opioid system is observed as a reduction in opioid receptor availability. Currently, it is assumed that these reductions might be related to competition of the endogenous transmitter with the radiolabelled ligand. However, they can also reflect other processes associated with the release of the endogenous neurotransmitter: a) receptor desensitization and internalization, b) ligand wash out due to stimulus-induced changes in regional blood flow, or c) a combination of all processes (Laruelle, 2000; Sprenger et al., 2005). In the first published [$^{11}$C]carfentanil study pain stimuli applied to the masseter muscles reduced μ-opioidergic binding in the dorsal anterior cingulated cortex, insula, thalamus, hypothalamus, amygdala and lateral prefrontal cortex (Zubieta et al., 2001). As hypothesized, subjective pain ratings correlated negatively with activation of the opioidergic system in the amygdala, thalamus and nucleus accumbens. Most importantly, this and other following ligand-PET studies (Bencherif et al., 2002; Casey, 1999; Ingvar, 1999; Sprenger et al., 2006; Zubieta et al., 2002) found activations in areas that are broadly consistent with those observed during functional imaging of acute pain (Casey, 1999; Ingvar, 1999). Thus, data suggests that μ-opioid-mediated analgesia not only takes place at the spinal dorsal horn level, but also in 'higher' brain areas and is involved in the individual experience of pain. Besides studies using experimentally induced acute pain in healthy volunteers, endogenous opioid neurotransmission is also being investigated in clinical pain states in chronic pain patients. Chronic inflammatory and neuropathic pain studies have found decreased binding of radiotracers in several key pain areas (Jones et al., 1994; Willoch et al., 2004). Interestingly, opioid neurotransmission normalized after reduction of pain symptoms, however not answering the issue of cause and effect. Or in other words, not solving the question: what came first, the hen or the egg? Future studies that correlate binding potential with pain intensity, could at least help elucidate whether decreased receptor availability is caused by increased release of endogenous opioids or decreased receptor density (Tracey and Mantyh, 2007).

## 2.3     Emotional and cognitive modulations of pain

Summing up, pain is a conscious sensory and emotional experience that arises from ascending and descending neural processing of a nociceptive input. Thereby, its perceived intensity and unpleasantness is not necessarily related linearly to the stimulus input, but is rather the result of genetic, pathological, and mental factors. It is important to note, that pain is often not only experienced as an intrusion to one's present body state, ease, or activity but also to one's future well-being and life in general. Distress about immediate threat and future implications, such as suffering due to persistency may intensify the pain experience and affect response priorities by catastrophic thinking and increased anxiety levels. Whether one's efforts are to escape, to endure, to reduce, or to avoid pain and pain-evoking situations is intrinsically related to one's momentary motivation and emotions. Naturally, these may change over an extended period of time as for example in chronic pain states (Ramirez-Maestre et al., 2008).

In recent years researchers have described several pain modulatory effects of mental processes. Especially the un-invasive access to the human CNS through neuroimaging tools have helped to understand how cognitive and emotional factors interact with descending pain modulatory circuits (Ingvar, 1999; Rainville, 2002; Tracey and Mantyh, 2007; Wiech et al., 2008b).

### 2.3.1 Attention, anticipation and expectation of pain relief

Attentional control of pain has extensively been studied (Villemure and Bushnell, 2002; Wiech et al., 2008b). Pain is perceived as less intense when somebody is distracted from it, as for instance by a cognitive task, and increases when attention is focused on it. The altered intensity ratings are accompanied by decreased activity in insula, thalamus, somatosensory cortices and anterior cingulated cortex (Bantick et al., 2002; Petrovic et al., 2000; Peyron et al., 1999; Valet et al., 2004). It has been postulated that distraction might at least partly act via opioid-mediated activation of descending pain modulatory systems (see chap. 2.2.3). Furthermore, attentional processes are closely related to expectations and emotions about pain and these in turn to prior experience. For instance, if the extraction of the first wisdom tooth was very unpleasant one might allocate even more attention during the extraction of the other three and consequently exacerbate the painful experience. A recent fMRI study elegantly showed how one's expectations strongly bias the interpretation of a noxious input. Expectation of a highly painful stimulus leads to increased anticipatory activation in pain-related brain areas and augments intensity ratings of subsequent pain (Koyama et al., 2005). Fortunately, the other way around is also effective: positive expectations diminish the severity of perceived pain and might be of therapeutical relevance for chronic pain states. Studies comparing dispositional optimism and pessimism affirm these findings. Individuals high in dispositional optimism, i.e. who tend to believe future outcomes will be positive, experience less pain when encountering a brief pain stimulus than pessimists (Geers et al., 2008).

The placebo effect, a well-known contextual influence on appraisal, can be taken as a model of a top-down regulatory process. Most remarkably, placebo analgesia, which is pain relief caused by the mere expectation of receiving an analgesic drug, can be blocked by the opioid receptor antagonist naloxone, implying an *exclusive* role of the endogenous opioid system (Levine et al., 1978).[8] Using state of the art molecular imaging techniques (see chap. 2.2.3) researchers confirmed that placebo analgesic effects are mediated by endogenous opioid activity on μ-opioid receptors (Benedetti et al., 2005; Zubieta et al., 2005). Data of a recent fMRI study supports the concept that prefrontal mechanisms can trigger opioid release within the brainstem during expectancy influencing the descending pain modulatory system and subsequently modulating pain perception (Wager et al., 2004). These findings are an intriguing example, how a complex mental activity, such as expectancy, interacts with different neuronal systems, mediating internal control of perceptual, motor, and homeostatic processes. In short, mental constructs, such as the context of beliefs and values, can trigger molecules that activate brain mechanisms in a similar way drugs do. These findings blur the line between pharmacodynamic and psychosocial drug effects and are continuously shaping our conception of how clinical trials and medical practice must be viewed and conducted (Colloca and Benedetti, 2005).

### 2.3.2 Perceived control

Pain is primarily perceived as a warning signal for threat of bodily integrity. Obviously, the degree of threat depends on the severity of the noxious drive. It is however also dependent upon one's momentary perception of control. The feeling of whether pain is in control of one's body and self, or if it is oneself that is in control and sufficiently able to cope with it, shapes the perceived pain intensity and unpleasantness. It is easier to endure pain when one is in control of the exposed amount of pain and particularly, is able to terminate the painful stimulus (Macdonald and Leary, 2005). For instance, removing a splinter is less painful when oneself is manoeuvring the needle, then when someone else is. Likewise, patients who are permitted to control their analgetic dose, as for example over a morphine infusion pump, need less analgetics and have shorter reconvalescence time after surgery (Wasylak et al., 1990). This effect is often integrated in pain treatments using patient-controlled analgesia (PCA), where patients are able to compensate for individual differences in metabolism and elimination of opioids. The analgetic effects of perceived control are even observed when the controlling response is only illusory, as for example when using a fake joystick response to reduce heat stimuli. Two years ago an fMRI study showed how perceived

---

[8] The observation that cognitive modulation of pain, as seen in anticipation of pain relief, is based on a single neurotransmitter system, will be contrasted to the investigations on emotional modulation of pain in the *opioid study* in chap. 6.4. Further critical discussion can be found on pp. 120–128.

control over a painful stimulus influences its neural response by a decrease in activity in anterior cingulate, insular, somatosensory cortices (Salomons et al., 2004). The observation that perceived controllability attenuates the aversiveness of a noxious input suggests a close relation to reappraisal processes. If one believes in being able to cope with a painful experience the following reinterpretation of emotional significance, i.e. reappraisal, decreases its perceived menace.

### 2.3.3 Reappraisal and perceived self-identity

Reappraisal is a powerful coping resource. The individual is constantly confronted with information from the internal and external world. According to his motivations, emotions and belief systems he has to select from diverse interpretation alternatives. Religion can be a very strong belief system and there are innumerable anecdotes of enduring pain through the power of religious belief. The emergence of powerful pharmacological analgetics has lead to a shift from suffering in the eye of religious belief to the ideal of a medicated painfree society. Still, there are many pain states, such as phantom limb pain or other chronic pain states, where pharmacological agents fail to help and spirituality is needed as before. Last year a British fMRI study investigated possible neural mechanisms underlying analgesic effects of religious belief (Wiech et al., 2008a). They postulate, that catholic participants contemplating on an image of the Virgin Mary were able to modulate their experience of pain through cognitive reappraisal of the negative emotional impact of pain via activity in the right ventrolateral prefrontal cortex (VLPFC).

Without doubt cultural background influences our approach and effort of dealing with life's challenges. It sets the personal standards for appraisal. In daily life we are used to adapt to different social systems by constantly and often naturally taking up positions and roles, as for example being a partner, sister, son, friend, lover, colleague, assistant, or leader. These roles are part of a certain value system, are often explicitly or implicitly hierarchical, and are always accompanied by a set of expectancies, rights and responsibilities. Therefore, they decisively influence behaviour tendencies in order to meet the demands and expectancies of the environment and particularly of oneself. Sport events are striking illustrations of how much pain an individual can endure in order to be respected. Depending on the rules and traditions of the sport, pain endurance changes its importance. While it is completely accepted or even expected that a soccer player wails in pain on the grass after being fouled, road racing cyclists seemingly gloat over their sufferance and self-endurance in front of the camera.[9] Thus, the perceived role, i.e. self-identity, in a certain context and social system governs the attribution of meaning to an event and may change its emotional impact. Thereby, it shapes appraisal and emotional response towards a positive or negative event such as pain.

In the study "**Perceived role-identity changes pain perception**" (see chap. 5) the impact of two opposing roles (*hero/heroine* and *faint-heart*) were investigated. Assuming that emotions may be elicited and augmented through the self-perceived role identity a change in subjective pain perception was expected. More specifically, it was hypothesized that (a) pain can be better tolerated whenever role identity is embedded in an unavoidable, unpleasant context, but which confers pain a meaningful and thus suitable character, and (b) that the self-perceived identity changes emotions accordingly, which in turn affects intensity and quality of pain perception.

### 2.3.4 Positive and negative emotions

Pain and emotion are closely intertwined. Most often pain causes negative emotions, such as fear, despair, annoyance, exhaustion and anger. Astonishingly, some pain stimuli may also trigger positive emotions, such as pleasure or pride during athletic performance, rituals, sex or eating spicy food. The latter ones however, essentially require a context of controllability and, needless to say voluntariness, to do so. Vice versa, also emotional state and mood have a significant impact on pain perception and ability to cope. For instance, chronic pain patients often react with maladaptive anxiety and fear of movement thereby exacerbating their pain state (Haythornthwaite and Benrud-Larson, 2000). Experimental studies in healthy volunteers have used diverse techniques to study the effects of induced emotional states on pain. These included pleasant erotic or family pictures (de Wied and Verbaten, 2001; Junghofer et al., 2006; Meagher et al., 2001; Wunsch et al., 2003), humorous, romantic or erotic film scenes (Weisenberg et al., 1998; Zillmann et al., 1996), pleasurable music (Roy et al., 2008; Whipple and Glynn, 1992), pleasant odours such as food, floral, greenery scents (Marchand and Arsenault, 2002; Villemure et al., 2003), or hypnosis (Rainville et al., 2005).

---

[9] Lance Armstrong, who won the "Tour de France" in 7 consecutive years, was recently quoted as follows: "Cycling is so hard, the suffering is so intense, that it's absolutely cleansing. The pain is so deep and strong that a curtain descends over your brain. (...) Once, someone asked me what pleasure I took in riding for so long. 'Pleasure?' I said. 'I don't understand the question.' I didn't do it for pleasure, I did it for pain." Further thoughts on the relationship between pain and pleasure on pp. 113–120.

There is general agreement that pleasant emotional states reduce pain perception, whereas unpleasant emotional states exacerbate it. Astonishingly, the neural and chemical mechanisms underlying these processes are hardly being explored. Neuroimaging studies investigating modulations of nociceptive processing in cortical and subcortical areas depending on emotional state are seldom (Villemure and Bushnell, 2002). What is more, contemporary affective neuroscience has been "somewhat preoccupied with the bad over the good" (Berridge, 2003). While extensive studies try to understand how the brain causes negative affect such as fear thereby modulating pain, it is quite unknown how the brain causes positive affective reactions such as pleasure. At the same time, the beneficial effects of positive emotional states on pain (i.e. pleasure-related analgesia) and its biological substrates have somewhat been disregarded.

### 2.3.5 Endogenous opioids and the regulation of pain and emotion

It is largely unknown, how neurochemical control systems modulate emotional states (Dolan, 2002), but an increasing amount of data allows for first assumptions. It has been suggested that painful and pleasant sensations – although, or precisely because being regarded as opposites – have the same underlying neural circuitry and chemistry (Leknes and Tracey, 2008). Particularly, endogenous opioid systems may be considered as an important neurochemical interface between pain and positive emotional states (Bodnar, 2008; McNally and Akil, 2002; Ribeiro et al., 2005). The role of endogenous opioids as substrates of pain and emotions has been investigated in separate studies that shall be briefly recapitulated in the following.

As described in chapter 2.2.3 ligand positron emission tomography (PET) studies were able to demonstrate that pain is associated with reductions in the in vivo availability of μ-opioid receptors, reflecting the activation of endogenous opioid systems. Especially in brain regions thought to be mainly involved in mediating the affective components of pain (rostral anterior cingulate cortex, insula) increased opioid activation was observed (Sprenger et al., 2006; Zubieta et al., 2001). Recently, the role of μ-opioid neurotransmission in attentional and cognitive modulation of pain has been investigated (Benedetti, 1996; Enck et al., 2008; Tracey and Mantyh, 2007; Wiech et al., 2008b). It appears that inhibition and facilitation of pain by context, expectancy or attention are at least partly mediated by an opioid-sensitive descending pain modulatory system and by direct effects of opioids in cortical nociceptive-related areas, such as the anterior cingulate cortex (Benedetti et al., 2005; Colloca and Benedetti,

2005; Petrovic et al., 2002; Scott et al., 2007; Wager et al., 2004; Zubieta et al., 2005; Zubieta and Stohler, 2009).

The mood-brightening effects of opiates have been known and used for millennia (Brownstein, 1993). After comprehensive research in mice (Burgdorf and Panksepp, 2006; Fields, 2007; Panksepp, 2003), gradually PET ligand-activation studies are examining the involvement of opioid neurotransmission in the regulation of emotional states in humans. Until now, possible alterations in opioidergic neurotransmission were tested during 'sadness' in grieving widows (Zubieta et al., 2003), and 'euphoric feelings' in healthy joggers (Boecker et al., 2008). Moreover, endogenous opioid systems appear to be essential in the hedonic response to pleasant sensory and emotional stimuli, mediating the experiences of 'wanting' and 'liking' in mice and men (Berridge, 2003; Gospic et al., 2008; Pecina, 2008). Even the hedonic experience of reward and loss of money is sensitive to blockade of μ-opioidergic neurotransmission (Petrovic et al., 2008).

Thus intriguingly, both painful and pleasant sensations are associated with the release of endogenous μ-opioids. However, until now studies have mostly explored the role of μ-opioid neurotransmission in both phenomena in isolation and not their interaction that we experience a good many times in everyday life, as for example when eating spicy food (Leknes and Tracey, 2008). The study "**Pleasure-related analgesia activates opioid-insensitive circuits**" investigated for the first time the interaction of both phenomena (see chap. 6). Considering the abovementioned findings, it was hypothesized that positive emotional states elicited by pleasant stimuli are associated with enhanced μ-opioidergic neurotransmission, contributing to alleviated pain perception. To study the role of endogenous opioids in the emotional modulation of pain perception, the μ-opioid-receptor antagonist naloxone was administered that temporarily reverses μ-opioidergic effects. In specific, it was investigated whether the blockade of μ-opioid receptors by an injection of 0.2mg/kg naloxone could be shown to (a) attenuate the hedonic response to pleasant emotional pictures and (b) reduce pleasure-related analgesia.

# 3
# Materials and Methods

This chapter gives a detailed description of the used materials and methods. The measurements of pain threshold and tolerance, autonomous body response and collection of subjective ratings are common techniques in experimental pain and emotion studies. The specific designs of each of the three experimental studies are delineated at the beginning of the respective chapters (see for *psychophysics study* p. 33, *role-identity study* p. 43, and *opioid* study p. 59).

## 3.1 Subjects

All studies were conducted according to the guidelines of the *"Declaration of Helsinki"* for the treatment of experimental subjects. Volunteers gave fully, written informed consent for the projects, which were approved by the local Ethics Committee and the Swissmedic respectively (*opioid study*). To exclude acute or chronic pain, other illnesses, allergies, or pharmacological biases through medication, as for example the intake of analgetics or psychopharmaceuticals, among volunteers, each participant was screened with a homemade questionnaire. Participants were also asked not to drink caffeinated or alcoholic beverages 6 hours prior to the experiment. Handedness was determined using standard handedness inventories (Chapman and Chapman, 1987; Oldfield, 1971).

## 3.2 Pain stimuli

In experimental pain studies standardized and safe pain stimuli are used. Pain is usually evoked by laser, heat, cold, peripheral arterial ischemia, or irritating substances applied to the skin, such as capsaicin. In this work heat stimuli were administered to the volar forearm using a 30 x 30-mm peltier device (Medoc, Ramat-Yishai, Israel; TSA-II) placed at 2/3 of the distance from wrist to elbow. Individual pain threshold was measured using the search method starting at 43°C: participants were asked to increase or decrease the magnitude of the heat stimulus by themselves to the point they felt it changing from "*hot*" to "*painful*" (in the *psychophysics* and *opioid study* the below described method of limits was used to assess pain threshold). Pain tolerance was determined by the method of limits: Participants were asked to stop the constantly increasing heat stimulus at the moment they could not stand the heat any longer. To avoid physical injuries the pain tolerance measurement stopped automatically at a maximal temperature of 52°C. In the *psychophysics study* two measurements starting at 32°C with a constant rise of temperature of 0.5°C/sec were averaged for pain threshold and pain tolerance, respectively. Pain tolerances in the *role-identity study* were calculated as an average of four measurements starting at 35°C with a constant rise of temperature of 0.6°C/sec. Finally, pain threshold and tolerances in the *opioid study* were determined as the average of three measurements starting at 35°C with a constant rise of temperature of 0.8°C/sec. In order to diminish visual distraction, participants were blindfolded or asked to close their eyes during the full length of pain measurements.

## 3.3  Emotional stimuli

In the *role-identity study* a simplified form a role-play game was used to implicitly induce the two antithetic role identities of a *hero/heroine* and a *faint-heart* and concomitant changes in emotional state. In the *opioid study* pleasant emotional pictures induced pleasant emotional states. In the *psychophysics study* no intentional emotional manipulation was used.

### 3.3.1  Role induction

For role induction in the *role-identity study*, role-plays inspired by the famous fantasy role-playing game Dungeons&dragons™ (Wizards of the Coast, inc., Washington, USA) were written. To improve role empathy of men and women, role identities were written gender-specific concerning the main character. At six different points in time, participants were given choices as to what to do or where to go within a labyrinth embedded in the story line, which was not affected by the different decisions. The story lines described the main character whose identity should be adopted. The *hero/heroine* role identity implied a winner image with strong personality and athletic build, and had the motivated task to save a princess. In contrast, the *faint-heart* character meant the role identity of a victim with weak personality, and no motivated task for his/her suffering at all. Both roles started as robber-knights attacked a kingdom.

While the *faint-heart* was threatened in his castle, the *hero/heroine* was on his way to liberate a princess. Both entered a fatal labyrinth. In contrast to the *hero/heroine* the *faint-heart* was violently forced into it, without any hope to escape. He resented his fate, and was plagued by fire, rats and vertigo. On his search for the princess, the *hero/heroine* overcame these dangers. Both characters ended up facing a guardian, who unjustifiably punished the *faint-heart* and offered a deal to the *hero/heroine*: He or she was free to escape with the princess, provided that he or she was willing to suffer for her.

All story lines and the control text[10] were spoken and recorded in a sound studio by a professional male speaker. They all had a total length of 13 minutes. The resulting sound files were machine finished using the software Garageband 2.0 by Apple Computer Inc., and played to the participants by means of speakers placed half a meter in front of them with and arbitrary but constant room-filling loudness.

### 3.3.2 Pleasure induction

For pleasure induction in the *opioid study*, a standardized selection of highly pleasant emotional stimuli from the International Affective Picture System (IAPS) was used (Lang et al., 2004). These pictures have robustly been shown to induce positive emotional states and pleasure-related analgesia (de Wied and Verbaten, 2001; Rhudy et al., 2008). For each trial a set of 15 pictures was selected (picture set 1 and 2). Care was given that both sets of pictures were equivalent in mean normative valence and arousal ratings for male subjects (*picture set 1*: valence mean (S.D.) = 7.58 (1.43), arousal mean (S.D.) = 6.56 (2.01); *picture set 2*: valence mean (S.D.) = 7.38 (1.39), arousal mean (S.D.) = 6.28 (2.00)). They consisted mainly of erotic (couples in erotic poses, nude females) and sports pictures. According to the motivational priming hypothesis by Lang and co-workers (Lang et al., 1990) erotic pictures, having great motivational-relevance, lead to strong appetitive system activation and arousal (Bradley et al., 2006).[11] In order to control for order effects the two picture sets were presented in counterbalanced order. The 15 pictures in each set were presented in randomized order for 6 s, followed by a white screen as a inter-picture interval of either 2 s or 12 s, resulting in a total duration of 180 s. Participants were asked to attentively watch

---

[10] http://presse.verwaltung.uni-muenchen.de//einsichten_buch/lebenswissenschaften/zwei.pdf (2004)
[11] The IAPS slide numbers for the two sets were as follows: *picture set 1*: erotic (4220, 4225, 4641, 4651, 4659, 4670, 4680), sports (5621, 5626, 8080, 8186, 8190, 8499), varia (2071, 8501); picture set 2: erotic (4250, 4599, 4611, 4652, 4653, 4658, 4660, 4695), sports (8170, 8185, 8200, 8370, 8496), varia (2303, 7330).

the pictures, let them sink in and to be open to imagine themselves being part of the shown situation. A practice trial of two pictures familiarized the participants with the type of pictures they were going to see. Pictures were presented on a 19'' monitor in approximately 70 cm distance to the participant.

## 3.4 Autonomic reactivity

In experimental studies autonomic body responses can be informative markers of emotional state. Skin conductance level, has consistently been shown to covary with subjective emotional arousal ratings (Lang et al., 1990) and the magnitude of an acoustically elicited startle eyeblink response has proved to be a reliable marker for the valence of an emotional state. Both autonomic reactions are hypothesized to reflect activation of underlying brain systems that respond to either appetitive or defensive motivations (Lang, 1995). In the *role-identity study* we investigated in collaboration with Meike Brockmann (a speech therapist) and Claudio Storck (ORL doctor) whether we could observe effects of changes in role-identity and emotional state on voice parameters.

### 3.4.1 Skin conductance level

Skin conductance level (SCL) was measured with a Varioport Measurement System (Becker Meditec, Karlsruhe, Germany), an 8-channel recording system. After filtering and a tenfold-amplification (Anti-Alias filter to cut off high frequencies), data were digitized (12 Bit resolution) and saved on a compact flash card. For measurements, one single channel was used. Channel parameters were set as follows: sampling rate 256 Hz, saving rate 16 Hz, range 0.1–100 µS and resolution of 0.001 µS. During SCL recordings, current across electrodes was held constant at 0.5 V by means of a 16 Bit-resolution unit. Before recording, the palm of the non-dominant hand was cleansed with distilled water and two Ag/AgCl electrodes (5 mm contact area diameter, Marquette Hellige Medical Systems, Freiburg, Germany) filled with lubricating jelly (SCL-Paste, 0.5 % NaCl, Becker Meditec, Karlsruhe, Germany) were placed adjacently on the hypothenar eminence of the palm.

SCL analyis in the *role-identity study*: In order to analyze peak amplitudes of the recorded skin conductance signals triggered by pain measurements, signal peaks were related to each one of the four pain tolerance stimuli (pre- and post every condition) by using the automatically recorded time as a marker, upon the participants' stopping of the pain stimulus. Peak amplitude was calculated by subtracting the value at the beginning of the rising phase of the recorded signal from the value at the apex of the same signal slope. Thereafter, the median corresponding to the four peak heights of the pain tolerance measurements were calculated and used for statistical analysis. In order to control for possible differences in skin conductance levels due to the role-specific adjustments of the characters of the story line, SCL of *heroines/heroes*, female and male *faint-hearts* were separately averaged throughout the role-playing story (including their pain-stimuli associated responses at the end). To correlate the average SCL of male and female participants of the same condition, the length of the first part of the female role-playing story was adjusted to the male story line. Due to detached electrodes, data of two participants (1 woman, 1 man) were excluded from SCL analysis.

SCL analyis in the *opioid study*: In order to analyze whether the arousal induced by pleasant stimuli was sensitive to naloxone, the autonomous emotional response to pleasure induction was assessed by means of skin conductance level. SCL raw data of each participant was amplified, dedrifted, rectified, and averaged throughout the picture viewing periods per block (180 s).

### 3.4.2 Startle eyeblink response

A higher organism reacts to a sudden unexpected stimulus such as a flash of light or a loud noise with a startle response. It's fastest and most stable component is the sudden closure of the eyelids. The eyeblink, which is a rapid contraction of the orbicularis oculi muscle, i.e. the muscle surrounding the eye, occurs reflexively 30-50 ms after the onset of an abrupt acoustic stimulus. The magnitude modulation of the eyeblink response can be measured with electromyography (EMG) and is a commonly used index for the valence of the emotional state of an organism. Several studies have shown that the magnitude of the eyeblink is enhanced during fear states and diminished in a pleasant emotional context (Lang et al., 1990). In the *opioid study* startle eyeblink responses were measured from the orbicularis oculi muscle beneath the left eye, using two 4 mm Ag/AgCl electrodes placed 1.5 cm apart and a signal ground electrode placed on the mastoid bone (Blumenthal et al., 2005). Startle responses were elicited by a 50 ms, 90 dB (A) burst of white noise, with instantaneous rise time, presented binaurally over Philips SBCHP195 headphones. In each block blink magnitudes of three startle probes presented during picture viewing were averaged; no responses were scored as zero magnitude blinks. Startle probes were presented 3000 ms after picture onset.

### 3.4.3 Voice measurement

In the *role-identity study* participants were asked to phonate the vowel /a/ at two different moments of each run: once right at the beginning of the run, and a second time close to the end of role-induction or control (scientific text, or silence). Voice signals were recorded by means of a personal computer using the "Göttinger Heiserkeitsdiagramm" (Rehder und Partner Medizintechnik, Hamburg). From the recorded voice signals only middle parts without voice onset and offset phase were used to obtain Fundamental Frequency (F0), Jitter (variation of F0) and Shimmer (variation of amplitude). Voice parameter analysis was carried out off-line after the experiment. Two participants (1 woman, 1 man) had to be excluded from the voice analysis-data, because their voices were strongly irregular and showed symptoms of functional voice disorders.

## 3.5 Subjective reports

The subjective dimension of emotions and pain is of very high interest in neurocognitive studies. Although questionnaires and subjective scales are often biased by the experimental and reporting situation, and are time lagged to the actual experience, they are important means to approach the first person perspective of subjects.

### 3.5.1 Subjective ratings of pain

After pain tolerance measurements participants were asked to give subjective pain ratings on two consecutive 10-cm visual analogue scales (VAS) (Price et al., 1983). In the first one, used to evaluate pain intensity, 0 indicated *"no pain"* while 10 represented the *"worst pain experienced"*. The second scale was used to assess pain unpleasantness, with 0 indicating *"neutral"* and 10 *"extremely unpleasant"*. In the *role-identity study* additionally the German version (Stein and Mendl, 1988) of the McGill Pain Questionnaire (MPQ) was applied (Melzack, 1975). The MPQ consists of different rated adjectives that describe sensory and affective dimensions of pain, such as stabbing, sharp, cramping, splitting, tiring-exhausting, and cruel-punishing. The rank values of the words chosen were added up to obtain a score for the sensory and affective subscales.

### 3.5.2 Subjective ratings of emotions and mood

In the *opioid study* a key question was whether positive emotional states were induced and whether naloxone altered emotional appraisal. After picture viewing participants were asked to rate the emotions they had experienced *while* watching the IAPS pictures on a computerized SAM (self-assessment manikin questionnaire). The questions for valence was: *"How pleasant or unpleasant were your feelings while watching the pictures?"* and for arousal: *"How arousing (German: intensiv) were your feelings while watching the pictures?"*. The SAM consists of two sets of five cartoon pictographs depicting different levels of emotional valence and arousal (Lang, 1980). Subjects were requested to click with the mouse on or between the figures. For each dimension ratings between 1 and 9 were yielded. Ratings were scored such that 9 represented a high rating on each dimension. Visually oriented scales using graphic character eliminate the majority of problems associated with semantic measures and are relatively 'culture-independent'. The manipulation check for emotional induction was conducted after the pain ratings in order to minimize possible demand or expectation effects (Meagher et al., 2001).

In order to assess the influence of naloxone on mood the Mehrdimensional Befindlichkeitsfragebogen (MDBF) (Steyer et al., 1997) was used at the beginning and end of each experimental session (*opioid study*). It included adjectives for the dimension *"feeling well versus not well"*, *"alert versus tired"* and *"calm versus aroused"*. The adjectives were for example: zufrieden, gut, unwohl, ausgeruht, schlapp, unruhig, and gelassen. For each dimensions ratings between 1 and 5 were recorded. Ratings were scored such that 5 represented a high rating on each dimension (i.e. well, alert and aroused). The two parallel versions of the questionnaire were given in counterbalanced order.

### 3.5.3 Subjective ratings of role empathy and meaningfulness

During the *role-identity study* further VAS and a home-made questionnaire were applied. Three VAS with end values of 0 indicating *"not at all"* and 10 *"very strong"* were used to assess for 1) meaningfulness to stand the pain, 2) the intensity of role empathy, and 3) the intensity of role empathy in comparison to acting or playing other role-plays. To asses whether the implicit character imbedded in the corresponding story line was truly captured, participants were asked to freely label the nature of the emotional state they experienced using single words or short phrases. 92% of the given adjectives were quoted in a standard German Synonyms' Dictionary (Duden,

2004). For further analyses, adjectives were then split into the three categories *"appropriate"*, *"antonym"* or *"strange"* to the role identity of a *hero/heroine* or *faintheart* facing pain. Category frequencies were expressed in percentages.

## 3.6 Statistical analysis

Unless indicated otherwise, data were calculated using repeated measurements analysis of variance (ANOVA). Post-hoc comparisons were performed using t-tests for dependent samples, p-values in the ANOVAs and t-tests were corrected using Greenhouse-Geisser or Bonferroni correction respectively. The significance level was set at $p<0.05$ for all statistical calculations other than post-hoc comparisons, which were corrected as stated above.

## 3.7 Medication

In the *opioid study* participants were randomly assigned to either the naloxone or control group. To ensure double-blind standards, during the experimental period (Jan–June 08) none of the involved persons (i.e. participant, experimenter, medical doctor, nurse) knew the identity of the administered sterile solution (produced by the Kantonsapotheke Zürich). The subjects of the naloxone group were administered naloxone hydrochloride (0.2mg/kg; concentration 1mg/ml), the subjects of the control group an equivalent volume of saline (0.9% NaCl) by a medical doctor (Jan von Overbeck). Similar naloxone dosages (8mg or 0.14mg/kg) have prior been shown to completely antagonize endogenous opioid-mediated analgesia in healthy volunteers (Amanzio and Benedetti, 1999; Amanzio et al., 2001; Benedetti, 1996; Bruehl et al., 2002). To prevent high stress levels of the participants during the experiment a nurse (Dana Briegel) inserted an intravenous catheter in the non-dominant arm bend before starting the experimental procedure.

### 3.7.1 Pharmacodynamic und pharmacokinetic properties of naloxone

Naloxone is a competitive μ-opioid receptor antagonist with a lower affinity at κ- and δ-opioid receptors (detailed pharmacological properties are discussed in chap. 7.1). Doses of up to 3mg/kg have shown no agonistic effects of naloxone (Hill, 1981). Naloxone (Narcan®) has first been approved by Swissmedic in December 1978. Until now, naloxone is clinically used (Naloxon OrPha®) to prevent or reverse the effects of natural or synthetic opioids including respiratory depression, sedation and hypotension (Figure 1).

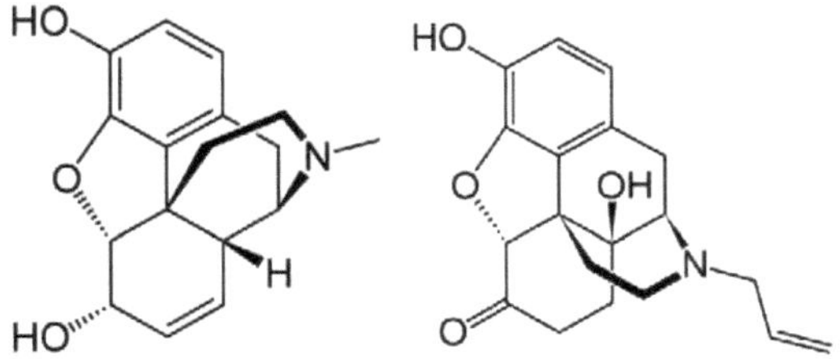

Figure 1: **Structural formulae of the μ-opioid receptor agonist morphine (left) and the μ-opioid receptor antagonist naloxone (right).**

Peak plasma levels in healthy volunteers have been measured 2 minutes after i.v. injection (0.01μg/ml). The onset of action is also generally apparent within 2 minutes after i.v. injection. Naloxone has a short serum half-life of around 70 minutes in adults (Arzneimittel-Kompendium, 2006). Adverse effects of naloxone in postoperative patients and subjects who are physically dependent on opioids are associated with abrupt reversal of opioid effects. Single doses of naloxone hydrochlorid of 10mg i.v., and cumulated doses of up to 90mg/d s.c., have shown no adverse effects or changes in laboratory values. According to the drug information of Narcan® the following side effects have been observed or can be potentially expected at very high doses of 2mg/kg (i.e. 140mg/70kg) in normal subjects (Narcan, 2001): cognitive impairment and behavioral symptoms (including irritability, anxiety, tension, suspiciousness, sadness, difficulty concentrating, and lack of appetite) and somatic symptoms (including dizziness, heaviness, sweating, nausea, and stomachaches). During the *opioid study* one participant reported dizziness at the end of the experimental session. The participant turned out to belong to the control group, thus the injected naloxone dose fortunately caused no adverse effects.

# 4

# Psychophysics of Pain

Quantification of experimental pain depends on the type of noxious stimuli used, their application and the assessment method: the stimuli are usually applied in fixed or ascending magnitudes, they can be assessed by threshold and tolerance measurements and subjectively characterized by pain ratings (Granot et al., 2006; Shy et al., 2003). It can be assumed that especially pain threshold and tolerance reflect the sensory experience provoked by a noxious stimulus more directly than subjective reports, because no time delay and no reflection veils the painful experience. A careful characterization of heat tolerance and threshold psychophysics at complementary sites oft the human forearm was an important starting point for my dissertation (Schaffner et al., 2008).[12]

## 4.1 Objectives and hypotheses of the study

Amongst others, heat pain tolerance measurements on the forearm have been proven to be a useful tool to investigate the effects of mental state (Bar et al., 2005; Bar et al., 2003) and gender (Fillingim et al., 1998) on pain perception. Therefore, the psychophysics of frequently used heat pain stimuli when applied to the forearms may provide a methodological basis for the growing number of psychophysical pain studies and might be of value for imaging studies on the laterality of brain dynamics during pain stimulation. No systematical evidence concerning pain thresholds and pain tolerance at different and homologous skin *sites* on the volar forearms has been presented so far, neither involving heat pain nor other noxious stimuli. To further characterize psychophysics of heat noxious stimuli, this study assessed whether varying the stimulus site on and across forearms may reveal equivalent pain threshold and toler-

---

[12] The study was published in August 2008 in *Neuroscience Letters* 440(3): N. Schaffner, A. Wittwer, E. Kut, G. Folkers, D.H. Benninger and V. Candia "Heat pain threshold and tolerance show no left-right perceptual differences at complementary sites of the human forearm". The first three authors contributed equally to the work.

ance values when randomly applied to either body side of healthy volunteers. These characterizations are important because there is a need for reference data of each body area, as Rolke et al. pointed out in seminal work (Rolke et al., 2006b). In particular, it was hypothesized that (a) pain tolerance and (b) threshold of heat noxious stimuli in three corresponding left and right forearms' sites of healthy volunteers will be equivalent.

## 4.2 Design and methods of the study

Eighteen healthy, right-handed volunteers, eight women and ten men, were recruited for the study. Mean age of participants was 35.2 years (S.D. 9.46). Noxious heat stimuli were randomly administered to six predefined *sites* within the volar aspect of the left and right anterior forearm. The time interval between the end of one stimulus and the start of the next stimulus was set at 10sec. The thermode was in contact with the skin approximately 5 seconds before stimulus commencement. On both forearms three homologous *sites* were individually assigned dividing the distance from wrist to elbow into equidistant segments. To check small perceptual variations resulting from variations in probe positioning (Price et al., 1989) the stimulus *sites* were marked on the skin with a water insoluble pen (see Figure 2). Pain threshold and pain tolerance were assessed for all *sites* in two separate measurement runs. Pain threshold was always measured prior to pain tolerance in order to avoid sensitization effects arising from longer stimulus duration of tolerance measurements, and counterbalance the fact that random paradigms in which intense stimuli immediately precede threshold measurements result in changed threshold estimates (LaMotte and Campbell, 1978). For comprehensive methodical description please see chap. 3.2.

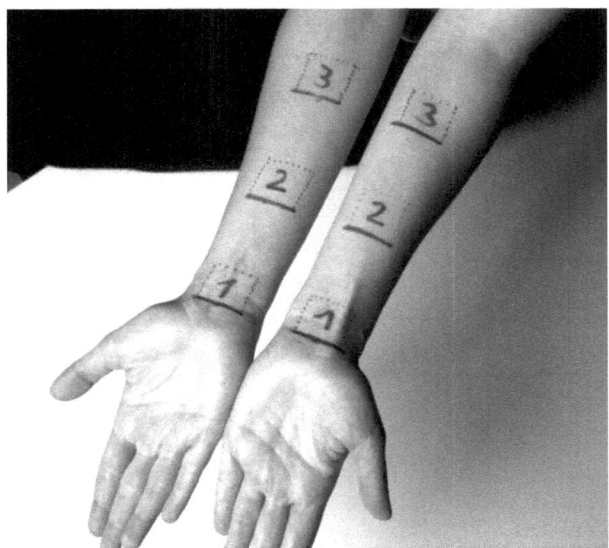

Figure 2: **Locations of the three stimulation *sites* on both forearms.**

### 4.2.1 Data analysis

To evaluate the effect of *site* and *side* of the body on pain threshold and pain tolerance a three factorial repeated measurements analysis of variance (ANOVA) with the factors *Site* (1-3), *Side* (right vs. left) and *Gender*, was calculated. In order to test for correlations amongst equivalent body parts, simple linear regressions were calculated. Two male participants exceeded the security limit set at 51°C, so that exact device readouts for their pain tolerance were not available. The security limit was arbitrarily assigned as their tolerance value. However these values were included only in the average gender comparisons.

## 4.3   Results

### 4.3.1 Pain threshold

The repeated measurements ANOVA for pain thresholds did not reveal any significant differences, neither in the main factors *Gender* ($F_{1,16} = 3.14$, $p = 0.096$), *Site* ($F_{2,32} = 1.66$, $p = 0.21$) and *Side* ($F_{1,16} = 0.32$, $p = 0.58$), nor in their interactions (See Table 2 for the average thresholds of all *sites* tested). Linear regression analysis revealed a significant relationship of pain threshold between averages from equivalent sites on the left and the right forearm (*Site 1 left vs. site 1 right:* $F_{1,16} = 30.48$, $|r|=0.81$, R Squared = 0.66, p < 0.0001; *site 2 left vs. site 2 right:* $F_{1,16} = 23.25$, $|r|= 0.77$, R Squared = 0.59, p = 0.0002; *site 3 left vs. site 3 right:* $F_{1,16} = 92.57$, $|r| = 0.92$, R Squared = 0.85, p < 0.0001, see Figure 3a).

Table 2: **Mean pain thresholds and pain tolerances (°C) split by gender.** Values are means and standard deviations (S.D.) for all three *sites* tested at the volar aspect of the right and left forearms. The numbers 1, 2 and 3 correspond to the stimulation *site* from wrist to elbow.

| Threshold | Right side | | | | Left side | | | |
|---|---|---|---|---|---|---|---|---|
| Forearm site | 1 | 2 | 3 | Mean (S.D.) | 1 | 2 | 3 | Mean (S.D.) |
| Males (n=10) | 45.77 (1.66) | 45.08 (2.70) | 44.89 (2.44) | 45.25 (2.17) | 45.44 (2.44) | 45.87 (2.24) | 45.28 (2.52) | 45.50 (2.33) |
| Females (n=8) | 43.51 (2.08) | 43.97 (1.21) | 43.80 (1.49) | 43.76 (1.50) | 43.92 (1.95) | 43.95 (1.66) | 43.42 (1.42) | 43.76 (1.61) |
| All (n=18) | 44.77 (2.14) | 44.59 (2.19) | 44.41 (2.09) | 44.59 (2.00) | 44.76 (2.31) | 44.97 (2.16) | 44.45 (2.26) | 44.73 (2.18) |
| Tolerance | | | | | | | | |
| Males (n = 10) | 49.03 (1.24) | 49.04 (1.86) | 49.00 (1.58) | 49.02 (1.51) | 49.03 (1.62) | 49.50 (1.75) | 48.91 (1.49) | 49.14 (1.56) |
| Females (n=8) | 47.41 (1.52) | 47.81 (0.72) | 47.72 (0.55) | 47.65 (0.79) | 47.39 (1.26) | 47.67 (0.91) | 47.49 (0.69) | 47.52 (0.85) |
| All (n=18) | 48.31 (1.57) | 48.50 (1.57) | 48.43 (1.37) | 48.41 (1.39) | 48.30 (1.66) | 48.69 (1.68) | 48.28 (1.38) | 48.42 (1.51) |

### 4.3.2 Pain tolerance

The repeated measurements ANOVA for pain tolerance including the factors *Gender*, *Site* and *Side*, revealed a significant main effect for the factor *Gender* ($F_{1,16} = 6.25$ p = 0.02): men showed higher pain tolerance for heat noxious stimuli than women (See Table 2 for the average tolerances of all *sites* tested). No other main effects or interactions were significant (*Site* ($F_{2,32} = 1.41$, p = 0.26) and *Side* ($F_{1,16} = 0.002$, p =

0.97). All computed regression analyses amongst averages of equivalent *sites* on the left and the right forearm were significant (*Site 1 left vs. site 1 right:* $F_{1,14} = 31.77$, $|r| = 0.83$, R Squared = 0.69, p <0.0001; *site 2 left vs. site 2 right:* $F_{1,14} = 24.66$, $|r| = 0.80$, R Squared = 0.64, p = 0.0002; *site 3 left vs. site 3 right:* $F_{1,14} = 38.90$, $|r| = 0.86$, R Squared = 0.74, p <0.0001, see Figure 3b).

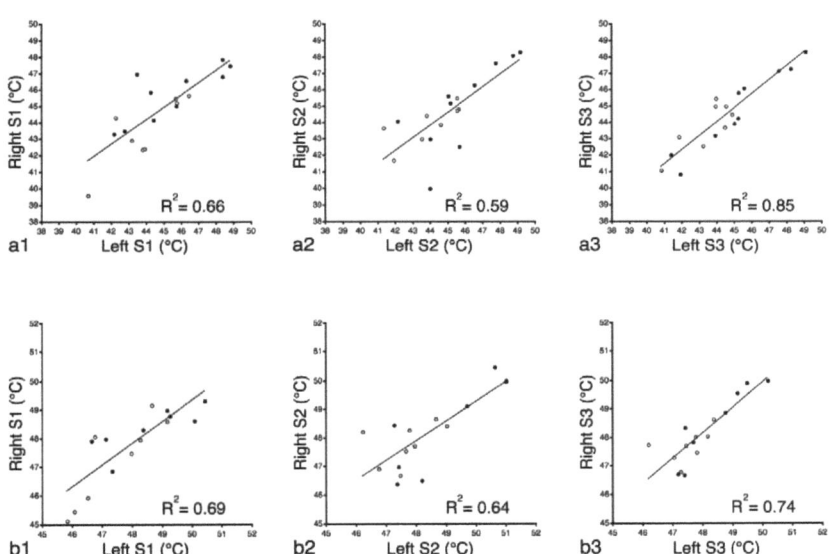

Figure 3: **Linear regressions of pain threshold (a) and tolerances (b) in °C between averages from equivalent *sites* on the left and the right forearms.** Depicted in the upper panel are regressions for pain thresholds at *sites* 1 (a1), 2 (a2) and 3 (a3). Shown in the lower panel are regressions for pain tolerances at *sites* 1 (b1), 2 (b2) and 3 (3b). S = *site*, filled dots = male subjects, unfilled dots = female subjects.

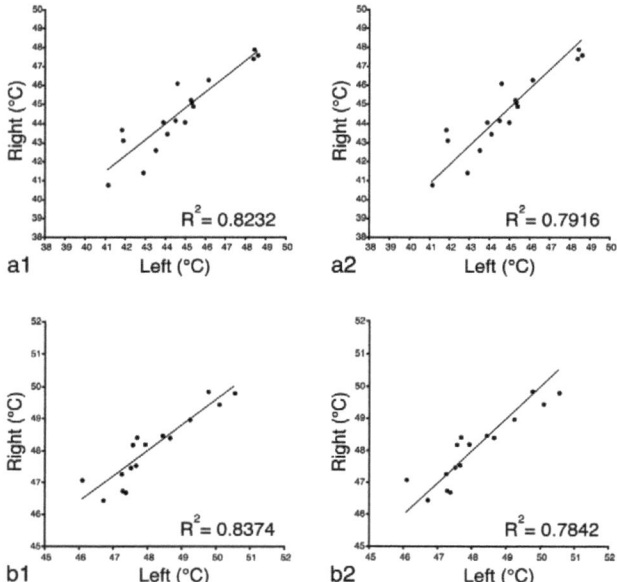

Figure 4: **Linear regressions of pain threshold (a) and tolerances (b) in °C, including averages from all sites on the left and the right forearms of all subjects.** Depicted in the left panel are regression lines showing the best linear fit (a1) and (b1) of a regression with unforced y-intercept. Shown in the right panel are regression lines with forced y-intercept crossing at zero (a2) and (b2). The results are similar irrespective of the fact that the y-intercept is forced to be zero or not. In addition, residuals do not reveal apparent outliers. Therefore, results appear to be valid at the individual level as well, and at least for heat pain thresholds and tolerances, laterality results do not appear to depend on stimulus intensity.

## 4.4 Discussion

In healthy volunteers, no perceptual differences in pain threshold and pain tolerance could be observed when heat pain stimuli were randomly applied to three different equidistant stimulus sites on the volar aspect of both forearms. These results were gender independent for pain thresholds and tolerances, though overall, men had higher pain tolerances.

On either side of the body we found equivalent thresholds for randomly applied heat pain stimuli for all three homologous sites. These results correspond to several studies using experimental heat pain stimuli reporting no side differences of thresholds on the forearm (Meh and Denislic, 1994; Spernal et al., 2003; Taylor et al., 1993) the hand (Yarnitsky et al., 1995) and the hand, foot and face (Rolke et al., 2006a; Rolke et al., 2006b). Concerning this absence of side effects on threshold, the study with the largest sample size was conducted by Rolke et al. (Rolke et al., 2006a). While some studies using tonic heat stimuli and subjective pain scores did not find left-right perceptual differences either (Long, 1994; Sarlani et al., 2003), others found higher pain perception of the left hand (Lugo et al., 2002). Studies using other painful stimuli than heat showed lower thresholds for electrical (Meador et al., 1998), pressure (Pauli et al., 1999) and cold (Schiff and Gagliese, 1994) stimuli presented to the left side of the body, but lower threshold for the dorsum of the right hand for heat noxious stimuli without tactile components (Schlereth et al., 2003). Several factors might explain these heterogeneous results concerning the effect of side on pain threshold. Laterality biases may strongly depend on the kind of noxious stimulation being used, resulting in the stimulation of different nociceptors with particular properties and impact on central mechanisms (Spernal et al., 2003). Some contradictory results regarding laterality of pain perception have also been obtained by using subjective pain ratings, such as visual analogue scales. Alternatively, differences in random vs. non-random stimulus presentation might explain the incongruence of these results. It is likely that an interaction of the above mentioned factors might have caused the observed differences.

In healthy volunteers and in patients, pain thresholds for heat pain stimuli have been analyzed for different parts of the body on one *side*, such as forearm, foot and hand (Kalter-Leibovici et al., 2001; Taylor et al., 1993; Yarnitsky et al., 1992). Mean receptor threshold for heat on receptive fields of C-nociceptors in the dorsum of foot and hand was found to be uniform (Yarnitsky et al., 1992). Significant differences in thresholds were found between glabrous and hairy skin *sites*, but not between the thenar eminence of the hand and the plantar surface of the foot (Taylor et al., 1993). Our results show for the first time that heat pain threshold *and* tolerance are highly similar across three different *sites* within the volar aspect of each forearm. These results add objective data to the findings of others who have observed that subjective ratings of supra threshold heat pain stimuli do not differ between *sites* within one forearm (Granot et al., 2003) or between thenar, volar and dorsal *sites* of the hand (Hagander et al., 2000).

The psychophysics of heat pain tolerance at different *sites* of the forearm has not been investigated so far, and only two studies have investigated the effect of body *side* at the volar wrist: in depressed patients, right hand *side* tolerance for thermal and electrical pain was increased whereas healthy controls showed no laterality effects

(Bar et al., 2005; Bar et al., 2003). The present results reveal that pain tolerance is not only equivalent on the volar wrists, but also on the other two equidistant *sites* on both forearms.

Several experimental and clinical studies on acute and chronic pain have shown that women are more sensitive to pain (Kuba and Quinones-Jenab, 2005; Rhudy and Williams, 2005; Rollman et al., 2004). In agreement with previous studies, our data show that overall, men have an higher pain tolerance than women for induced heat pain (Fillingim et al., 1998; Kut et al., 2007). Similarly we did not observe a gender difference in pain threshold, only a light tendency ($p=0.096$), although the small number of subjects may have obscured a possible difference. A power analysis including a power value of 0.80 and a difference in heat pain threshold between genders of 1.62°C, with a joint sigma value of 2.04, revealed that a sample size of 25 volunteers for each sample would be needed to achieve a significant gender effect. This should be considered for a gender difference study in the future. Concerning heat pain threshold existing data are controversial: in 180 patients Rolke et al. found gender differences (Rolke et al., 2006a) while others observed no gender effect (Kut et al., 2007; Yosipovitch et al., 2004).

Some limitations of our data should be considered. Given the large influence of age on thermal thresholds including older subjects (the oldest participant included was 43 years old) might reveal different outcomes for the measured perceptual parameters (Rolke et al., 2006a). In addition, our sample included only 18 subjects. Though, our sample size is similar to those in other studies on pain perception that used a comparable methodology (Rolke et al., 2006b). Differences in thermode pressure against the skin were not controlled in any special way. This factor has been discussed to be a potential confound in similar pain measurement setups. The strong relationships we observed suggest that slight pressure differences do not significantly affect position-temperature relationships, at least amongst homologous body locations.

Regression lines for thresholds and tolerances show that the y-intercept is slightly – but consistently – positive (see Figure 3). This may suggest that psychophysical outcomes on laterality would depend on the physical intensity of the stimulus. By computing a simple regression including the left and right averages over all *sites* of any single subject, a high linear fit for both, tolerances and thresholds is again obtained. Results are highly similar, irrespective of the fact that the y-intercept is forced to be zero or not. In addition, residuals do not reveal apparent outliers (see Figure 4). Therefore, the results appear to be valid at the individual level as well, and at least for heat pain thresholds and tolerances, laterality results do not appear to depend on stimulus intensity.

The high correlations of threshold and tolerance values across *sites* and *side* of stimulation suggest a rather evenly distributed density of heat pain receptors amongst the *sites* in the forearms. Different receptor densities across pain receptive fields would probably lead to differences in threshold and tolerance values. As has been demonstrated in the forearms of monkeys, the heat threshold and the response magnitude at suprathreshold intensities depends on the size of the skin area overlapped by the heat stimulus (Treede et al., 1990). Infrared-recorded thermal imprints of our heat stimuli on both forearms of a volunteer not included in the present series cover an equivalent skin area (see Figure 5).

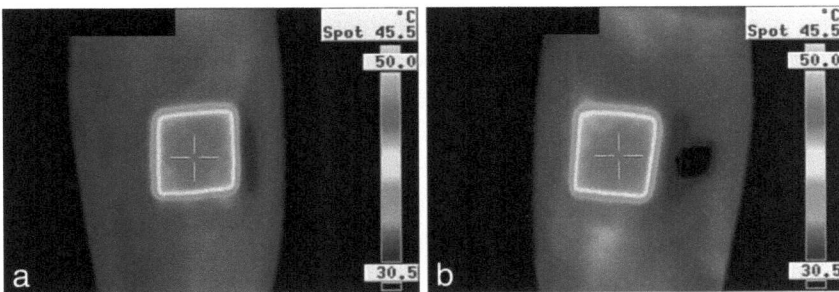

Figure 5: **Infrared thermogram on right forearm (a) and left forearm (b) of a volunteer not included in the present series captured immediately after stimulation with a fixed temperature.** Note that the thermal imprints cover an equivalent skin area, and the effect of the stimulus remains local. The dark area right below the thermode originates from the coolant hose of the system [ThermaCam PM545, FLIR, Danderyd, Sweden. Thermal sensitivity <0.1°C at 30°C; Spectral range 7.5–13 µm; built-in digital video 320×240 pixels.].

Some recent brain imaging studies have reported right brain lateralization for the processing of electrical pain stimuli (Symonds et al., 2006). In contrast, other studies using laser stimulation, which is selective for the stimulation of nociceptors, have clearly shown a significant contralateral bias within the somatosensory cortex for stimulation of either hand (Bingel et al., 2003) and the legs (Youell et al., 2004).

Whether results would be different in patients remains an open issue. It is an interesting question to what extent this technique might be discriminative for focal or distal sensory deficits. For example, left-right differences might be observed in patients with focal lesions while *site*-to-*site* differences in patients suffering from polyneuropathy. In addition, the magnitude of *side* and *site* differences, which may be considered to be within normal limits, in single individuals, should be clarified in future work.

## 4.5 Conclusion

A growing body of psychophysical pain studies operates with pain threshold and tolerance as objective measures to investigate effects of mental state on pain. Amongst other types of noxious stimuli, heat pain tolerance measurements on the forearm have been proven to be useful and easily practicable. Since no systematical evidence concerning pain thresholds and pain tolerance at different and homologous skin sites on the volar forearms has been presented so far, this study set out to investigate, whether varying the stimulus site on and across forearms reveals equivalent pain threshold and tolerance values when randomly applied to either body side of healthy volunteers. Pain threshold and pain tolerance did not differ within and across forearm sites. Thus, experimenters addressing heat pain threshold and tolerance in healthy volunteers may freely choose and change stimulation sites on both volar forearms, without the risk of confounding site effects on dependent variables. Moreover, this data completes previous reports on side effects by analyzing the effect of site on the forearm for both heat pain threshold and tolerance. The absence of side and site effects may contribute to setting a more secure basis for assessments of laterality effects of painful stimulation. Within the scope of my dissertation, this study set the methodological basis for the pain measurements in the succeeding *role-identity* and *opioid studies*.

# 5
# Role-identity and Pain

The scenery in the two paintings of the Napolitano Gaspare Traversi (1732–ca.1769), are strikingly similar (see Figure 6) but to the attentive observer, they vividly depict opposing pain sensations in the face of the suffering patient: forced and on his own, he grimaces with intense pain, yet facing the proximity of a comforting woman he bravely and calmly endures the awful medical intervention. Apparently, the man perceives himself differently, and this changes his tolerance for the excrutiating pain.

In daily life we are used to adapt to different social systems by constantly and often naturally taking roles. These roles are part of a certain value system and decisively influence appraisal and behaviour tendencies in order to meet the demands and expectancies of the environment and particularly of oneself. Thus, the perceived role, i.e. self-identity, in a certain context and social system governs the attribution of meaning to an event and may change its emotional impact. The investigation of such changes in appraisal, sense-making and emotional response to pain was the aim of the following study (Kut et al., 2007).[13]

---

[13] This study was published in September 2007 in *Pain* 131(1–2): E. Kut, N. Schaffner, A. Wittwer, V. Candia, M. Brockmann, C. Storck, G. Folkers "Changes in self-perceived role identity modulate pain perception." In October 2007 the study was awarded with the "Förderpreis für Schmerzforschung 2007" of the Deutsche Gesellschaft zum Studium des Schmerzes e.V. (DGSS). The first three authors contributed equally to the work.

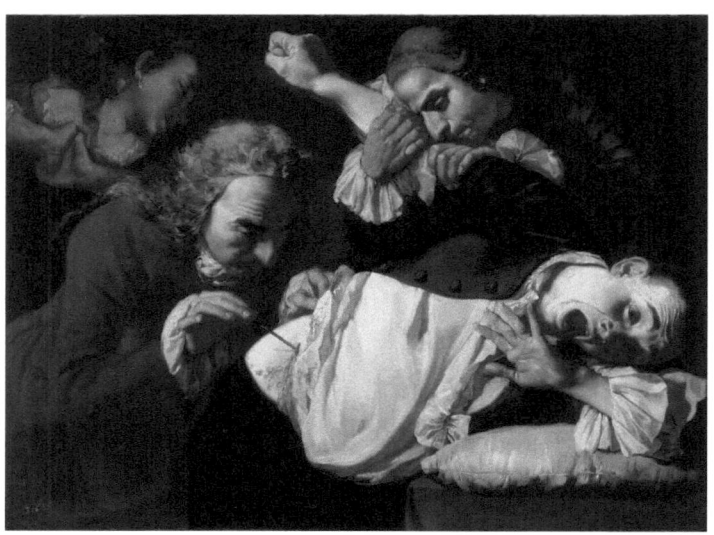

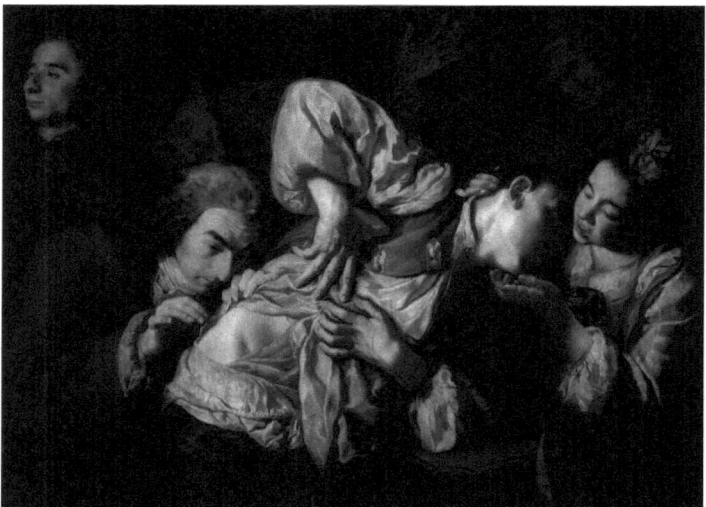

Figure 6: **Two paintings of the Napolitano Gaspare Traversi depicting opposing pain sensations.**
(Above) The suffering patient, when forced and on his own grimaces with intense pain. *"L'operazione chirurgica"* reproduced with permission of the Staatsgalerie Stuttgart. (Down) Comforted by a woman, he endures the awful procedure. *"Il Ferito"* reproduced with permission of the Gallerie dell'Accademia di Venezia. © 1990 Photo SCALA, Florence – courtesy of the Ministero Beni e Att. Culturali.

## 5.1 Objectives and hypotheses of the study

So far, the effect of self-perceived role identity on pain perception has only been investigated in gender role studies. Hereby, the effect of different, probably culturally induced, gender-role factors on pain have been shown. For example, coping strategies (Keogh and Herdenfeldt, 2002), pain catastrophizing (Thorn et al., 2004), situational context (Kallai et al., 2004), gender role expectations (Robinson et al., 2001) or anxiety (Edwards et al., 2000) have been studied. Besides gender roles, there are several more roles that shape appraisal, emotional state and action tendencies of an individual. In everyday life experiences different self-perceived role identies are known that enable to tolerate pain more easily. For example, parents very often encourage their children to transitorily adopt a brave and strong attitude in order to diminish unpleasantness during a painful medical intervention aimed at protecting them from or alleviating a distressing illness. Thus, understanding the alleviating power of a vaccination and empathizing with an archetype, which has the implicit ability to tolerate danger and to overcome pain can transform the painful procedure into a meaningful and tolerable experience. The use of this simple strategy may not be limited to childhood, but is most probably used during acute painful situations throughout life.

In this study, it was assumed that emotions may be elicited and augmented through the self-perceived role identity. More specifically, it was hypothesized that (a) pain can be better tolerated whenever role identity is embedded in an unavoidable, unpleasant context, but which confers pain a meaningful and thus suitable character, and (b) that the self-perceived identity changes emotions accordingly, which in turn affects intensity and quality of pain perception. In order to benefit from the strong identification effect during games (de Quervain et al., 2004; Singer et al., 2006), and in contrast to other emotion induction techniques, a simplified form of a role-playing game was used. The ultimate goal was to establish a learnable self-perceived role identity that can be of potential use in new pain management strategies.

## 5.2 Design and methods of the study

Twenty-one healthy volunteers experienced in assuming roles, either by regularly playing role-playing games or acting on stage, were recruited for the study. Mean age of participants was 28.2 years (S.D. ±10.0). Ten women (mean age 31.2 years, S.D. ± 12.7) and nine men (age 24.9 years, S.D. ± 4.5) were included in the study. Two participants were excluded from all data analyses because their pain tolerance exceeded the security limit set at 52°C.

In an experimental session, each participant underwent three different conditions: two role conditions (*hero/heroine* and *faint-heart*) and one control condition (sientific text *or* ten minutes silence without any other accompanying task). Conditions were presented to every study participant at random and in counterbalanced order. During the experiment participants lay on a couch in half-lying position but still were able to easily read the instructions displayed in a monitor placed at an arbitrary, yet constant distance in front of them. The experimenter affixed the thermode and the electrodes for SCL-recording. Thereafter participants were instructed on how to self-control the delivery of the painful stimuli by using two response buttons connected to the TSA-II. In addition, two different acoustic signals indicated either a tolerance or a threshold measurement. Participants were blindfolded with an appropriate mask for the full length of the experiment, except for the periods in which they had to complete a questionnaire. An experimental session consisted of three runs comprising both roles and one of the control conditions (see Figure 7).

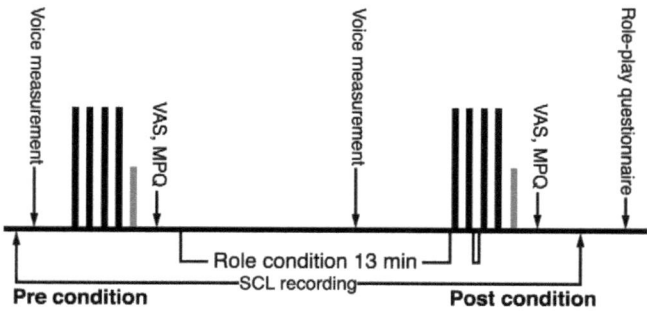

Figure 7: **Schematic depiction of an experimental run.** A break of five minutes was inserted between runs. Solid black bars represent the use of noxious heat stimuli for pain tolerance measurements, grey bars for pain threshold measurements respectively. The unfilled white-bar, in the middle of the second pain tolerance measurement, represents the continuation of the story line to avoid vanishing of the possible effects resulting from role induction procedures. VAS = visual analogue scale; MPQ = McGill pain questionnaire; SCL = skin conductance level.

At the beginning of each run, participants' voice signal was recorded followed by pain tolerance first, and then pain threshold measurements. Subsequently, subjective ratings concerning pain tolerance were collected. Thereafter, a role-playing story, the scientific text *or* the silent condition followed. Eight minutes after the start of a condition, the second voice measurement was carried out. Pain tolerance and pain threshold were both measured a second time immediately at the end of any condition. In order to sustain the role-identity effects during pain measurements, the role-playing story continued for 25 seconds after the first two stimuli of the second series consisting of four pain stimuli. Time interval between the four pain stimuli was always held constant and there was no overlap between listening periods and pain stimuli. After voice, pain tolerance and pain threshold measurements, subjective pain ratings were again collected. Subsequent to both role conditions the questionnaire concerning role empathy was completed. After five minutes rest a new run was started. To control for confounding factors associated to circadian variations, all participants were tested starting either at 5 pm or 6 pm. The total duration of an experimental session was approximately two hours. Volunteers were debriefed after the three experimental runs were completed, and they received a monetary compensation for their participation in the study.

### 5.2.1 Data analysis

The data of ten women (9 right-handed, 1 left-handed), and nine men (8 right-handed, 1 left-handed) were included in the analyses. First results of the control conditions 'scientific text' (n = 10, 5 women, 5 men) and 'silence' (n = 9, 5 women, 4 men) were compared with a one factorial repeated measurements analysis of variance (ANOVA) involving the factor *Time* (pre vs. post). Values of pain measurements, vocal and SCL recordings, as well as subjective reports did not show significant differences among the two control conditions. Thus, both, the "scientific text" and "silence" control groups were merged into a single control group for further comparisons. To evaluate the effect of role induction on pain tolerance and threshold, VAS ratings of pain intensity unpleasantness, and on the sensory and affective subscales of the MPQ repeated measurements analyses of variance with the factors *Role* (hero/heroine, faint-heart and control), *Time* (pre/post) and *Gender* were separately calculated. Post-hoc comparisons were made by means of paired single t-tests. To assess for the effect of time (Run1/Run2/Run3) on pain intensity and pain unpleasantness, a one factorial repeated measurements ANOVA on the scores resulting from the arithmetic addition of pre- and post-role induction in any of the three runs was calculated. To assess for changes in participant's emotional status during and after role induction, voice measurements, skin conductance level and role-play questionnaires were again evaluated by means of ANOVAS and Spearman's Rank correlations. Significance level (p) was set at 0.05 for all statistical calculations. For post-hoc t-test comparisons, the significance level was adjusted using the simple Bonferroni correction by dividing 0.05 by the number of possible single multiple comparisons in the corresponding effect (i.e. alpha-corrected: 0.003 for the *Role*Time* interaction and alpha-corrected: 0.016 for the *Time* effect (Run1/Run2/Run3) in the VAS ratings).

## 5.3     Results

### 5.3.1  Pain tolerance and threshold

The ANOVA for pain tolerance was significant for the main factor *Role* ($F_{2,17}$ = 9.58, p = 0.001). Most importantly, the interaction *Role*Time* was highly significant ($F_{2,17}$ = 21.46, p = 0.000; Figure 8). Post-hoc t-tests showed that pain tolerance increased significantly with the induction of the *hero/heroine* role ($t_{18}$ = -3.70, p = 0.002), however it significantly decreased in the case of the *faint-heart* role ($t_{18}$ = 3.87, p = 0.001). Listening to a scientific text or ten minutes silence without any other task led to a significant decrease in pain tolerance as well ($t_{18}$ = 4.49, p = 0.000). The interaction *Role*Gender* was not significant ($F_{2,17}$ = 1.57, p = 0.229). Overall, men showed higher pain tolerance than women ($F_{1,17}$ = 5.44, p = 0.032; Figure 9). In contrast to pain tolerance, pain threshold measurements did not significantly differ in any of the main factors or their interactions. Corrected alpha level for post-hoc t-tests: 0.003.

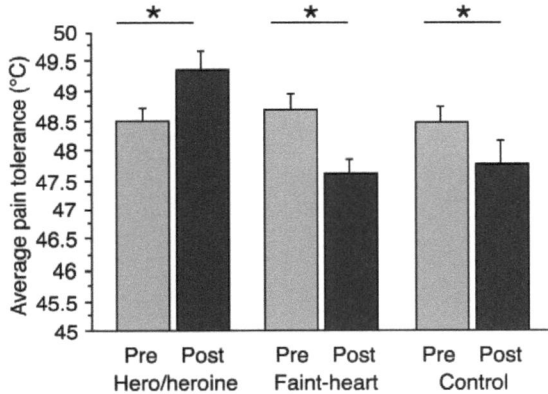

Figure 8: **Mean levels of pain tolerance (°C) pre- and post role induction and control conditions.** Asterisks (*) indicate significant, post-hoc comparisons (p < 0.003). Pre = pre-role induction/control conditions; Post = post-role induction/control conditions. Bars depict average values and standard errors.

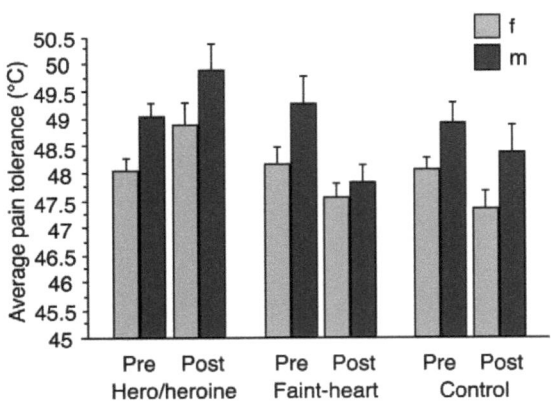

Figure 9: **Difference in pain tolerance between men and women.** Overall, men showed higher pain tolerance than women. Pre = pre-role induction/control conditions; Post = post-role induction/control conditions; f = females; m = males. Bars depict average values and their standard errors.

## 5.3.2 McGill pain questionnaire (MPQ)

The ANOVA for the sensory subscale of the MPQ was significant for the interaction Role*Time ($F_{2,17}$ = 9.24, p = 0.002). Post-hoc t-tests revealed that only *heroes/heroines* increased their sensory pain ratings significantly ($t_{18}$ = -4.04, p = 0.001;

Figure 10a). The ANOVA for the affective subscale of the MPQ was significant for the interaction *Role\*Time* as well ($F_{2,17} = 6.46$, p = 0.005). The post-hoc comparisons revealed that only *faint-hearts* significantly increased their affective pain ratings ($t_{18} = -3.58$, p = 0.002; Figure 10b). Overall, female volunteers gave higher MPQ ratings than men (sensory: $F_{1,17} = 11.40$, P = 0.004; affective: $F_{1,17} = 7.46$, p = 0.014). Control conditions showed no significant change in sensory and affective subscale scores. Corrected alpha level for post-hoc t-tests: 0.003.

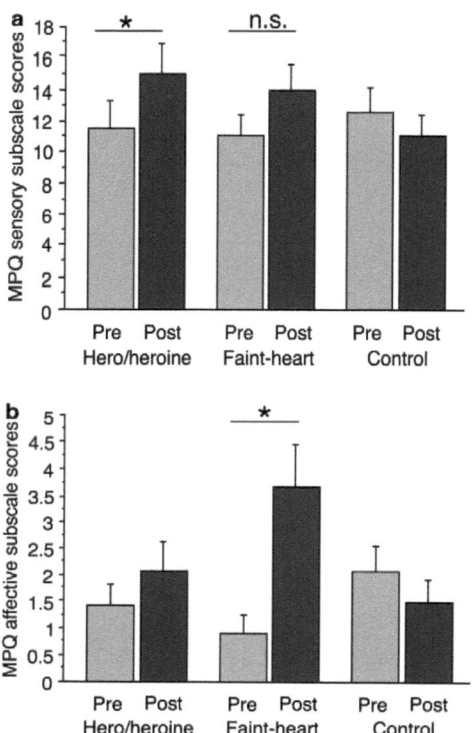

Figure 10: **Mean MPQ subscale scores pre- and post role induction and control conditions.** (a) Sensory subscale scores increased significantly only after the role induction of a *hero/heroine*. (b) Affective subscale ratings increased significantly only after the role induction of a *faint-heart*. Asterisks (*) indicate significant post-hoc comparisons (p < 0.003). Pre = pre-role induction/control conditions; Post = post-role induction/control conditions. Bars depict average values and standard errors.

### 5.3.3 Visual analogue scale (VAS) for pain intensity and unpleasantness

The ANOVA for the VAS on pain intensity ratings was significant for the interaction *Role\*Time* ($F_{2,17} = 3.94$, $p = 0.032$). Post-hoc t-tests showed a significant increase of pain intensity ratings for *heroes/heroines* ($t_{18} = -4.04$, $p = 0.001$). Neither role nor control conditions altered VAS ratings for pain unpleasantness. The ANOVA for the effect of time (Run1/Run2/Run3) on pain intensity was significant ($F_{2,17} = 3.66$, $p = 0.047$) as well as the corresponding ANOVA for pain unpleasantness ($F_{2,17} = 8.01$, $p = 0.004$): over time, scores on both measures increased. Nevertheless, post-hoc t-tests of pain intensity scores did not survive Bonferroni corrections. Conversely, mean pain unpleasantness ratings increased significantly from Run1 to Run3 ($t_{18} = -3.30$, $p = 0.004$). Corrected alpha level for post-hoc t-tests: 0.003 and 0.016 respectively. Women gave significantly higher pain unpleasantness ratings than men ($F_{1,17} = 4.99$, $p = 0.039$).

### 5.3.4 Role-play questionnaire

The ANOVA for VAS ratings for pain meaningfulness was significant for the main factor *Role* ($F_{1,17} = 12.40$, $p = 0.003$). Pain had more meaning for *heroes/heroines* than for *faint-hearts*. Conversely, the factor *Gender* was not significant as well as any interaction. The nonparametric Spearman Rank correlation revealed a significant correlation between the increase in pain tolerances of *heroes/heroines* (differences *post-pre*) and their corresponding VAS ratings on meaningfulness of pain collected at the end of the role induction (rho = 0.569, $p = 0.011$). We found no such correlations for *faint-hearts* (rho = -0.167, $p = 0.495$). VAS ratings on role empathy at the end of role induction of *hero/heroine* (71.4±21.8 S.D.) and *faint-heart* (65.3±22.3 S.D.) did not differ significantly from each other ($F_{1,17} = 0.03$, $p = 0.862$). Gender had no impact on role empathy either ($F_{1,17} = 2.92$, $p = 0.106$). In addition, the repeated measurements ANOVA for VAS ratings of the intensity of role empathy during the experimental procedure compared to during normal role-playing games showed no significant difference for the main factors *Role* ($F_{1,17} = 0.41$, $p = 0.53$) or *Gender* ($F_{1,17} = 0.61$, $p = 0.447$); (*heroes/heroines:* 56.6±25.5 S.D., *faint-hearts*: 60.5±20.2 S.D.). Freely chosen words or phrases at the end of each role condition indicating whether the implicit character imbedded in the corresponding story line was truly captured were mostly appropriate to the role identity of a *hero/heroine* or a *faint-heart* facing pain. In the *hero/heroine* condition 58% of the adjectives belonged to the category *"Appropriate"*, whereas 27% were *"Antonyms"* to the role identity of a *hero*. The remaining

15% were *"Strange"* adjectives. In the *faint-heart* condition 89% of the adjectives fell into the category *"Appropriate"* and 11% into the category *"Strange"*. At the end of the experimental session, participants reported no significant preference in having empathized with one role or the other: 3 men and 4 women preferred the *hero/heroine* identity, 4 men and 2 women preferred the *faint-heart* identity, while the remaining 6 reported they have equally empathized with both roles.

### 5.3.5 Autonomic responses

Both skin conductance levels (SCL) of *heroines* and *heroes* and SCL of female and male *faint-hearts* correlated highly significant (rho= 0.824, p = 0.000 and rho = 0.662, p = 0.000 respectively). Moreover, same signal traces of *heroines* and *heroes* together significantly correlated with those of *faint-hearts* (rho = 0.787, p = 0.000; Figure 11). The repeated measurements ANOVA for stimulus-related peak height of SCL during pain tolerance measurements was highly significant for the interaction Role*Time ($F_{2,15}$ = 17.72, p = 0.000). Post-hoc t-tests showed that the induction of the *hero/heroine* role lead to increased stimulus-related SCL peaks ($t_{16}$ = -4.33, p = 0.001), whereas the test results of *faint-hearts* and control conditions did not alter stimulus-related SCL peaks at all (*faint-heart*: $t_{16}$ = 2.75, p = 0.014; control: $t_{16}$ = 0.97, p = 0.346). Corrected alpha level for post-hoc t-tests: 0.003.

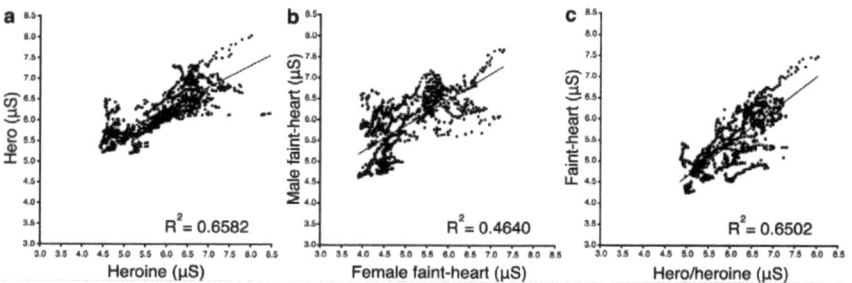

Figure 11: **Correlations of SCL of different roles and genders.** SCL were correlated from the start of a role induction up to and including the pain stimuli at the end of the role induction. Both SCL of *heroines* and *heroes* (a) and SCL of female and male *faint-hearts* (b) correlated highly significant. Moreover, same signal traces of *heroines* and *heroes* together significantly correlated with those of *faint-hearts* (c).

### 5.3.6 Voice measurement

The repeated measurements ANOVA for the voice measurements with the factors *Time*, *Role* and *Gender* revealed highly significant differences of Fundamental Frequency (F0) for the factor *Gender*: men showed lower F0 ($F_{1,15} = 59.12$, $p = 0.000$). Jitter (variation of F0) and shimmer (variation of amplitude) of participant's voices were not significantly different under any of the measured conditions (*hero/heroine*, *faint-heart*, control).

## 5.4 Discussion

In this study, the influence of self-perceived role identity, and its resulting emotional status on both, subjectively and objectively assessed pain was investigated. Role-play strategies were used to implicitly induce the two antithetic role identities of a *hero/heroine* and a *faint-heart*.

*Heroes/heroines* tolerated more heat and gave these stimuli higher pain scores in the sensory subscale of the MPQ. Nevertheless, associated affective pain ratings were not altered. Similarly, *heroes/heroines* showed higher pain intensity VAS ratings and unchanged pain unpleasantness scores. The experimental setting does not permit to clarify to which extent this role-identity caused the unchanged affective pain ratings. Another experimental design using constant stimuli may help to elucidate this effect. Most remarkably, *faint-hearts* showed higher affective MPQ ratings at lower temperatures and less pain tolerance. Only *faint-hearts* revealed significant affective MPQ scores, suggesting that this identity can amplify affective components of pain sensation. For every participant one out of two conditions was chosen to control for the effects of listening to a spoken text, answering questions, and for the speaker's voice. Pain tolerance was comparably lower after the *faint-heart* and control conditions. It is probable that hearing a hardly understandable scientific text or waiting blindfolded without knowing what will happen next led to unpleasant affective states promoting a low pain tolerance. In addition, MPQ and VAS scores for control conditions remained unchanged. Therefore, only a change in self-perceived role identity resulted in measurable differences in the perception of pain intensity and quality together with pain tolerance.

In addition, the influence of self-perceived role identity and its resulting emotional dimension *"arousal"* on acoustic vocal parameters and on skin conductance level (SCL) was assessed. SCL of participants correlated during both role-playing stories and did not differ between genders (Figure 11); this suggests similar levels of attention throughout role conditions. Higher stimulus-related SCL peaks after the *hero/heroine* role induction most probably resulted from the increased pain sensation at higher temperatures. Since stimulus-related SCL peaks did not decrease in the *faint-heart* and control conditions, it can be concluded that participants indeed stopped the pain stimuli at lower heat temperatures due to truly role-induced decrease in pain tolerance, and not due to, for example, differences in motivation. In contrast to previous reports (Johnstone and Scherer, 2000; Mendoza, 1998), the results of vocal parameters did not allow for final conclusions. Probably, lack of sensitivity and specificity (Ludlow, 1987; Zyski, 1984), amongst others, may explain the results.

Anticipation of pain influences pain sensation, and anticipatory coping mechanisms have been discussed (see chap. 2.3.1) (Hsieh et al., 1999; Ploghaus et al., 1999). Every pain measurement was announced by means of a consistent auditory signal. Therefore, anticipatory effects can be assumed to similarly affect all the conditions used. The diverging results for the antithetic self-perceived role identities do not support anticipatory mechanisms.

Role and control conditions did not alter VAS unpleasantness scores. However, these scores increased over time of the experiment, presumably as a result of the repeated noxious stimuli. Because VAS pain scores of heat pain have been shown to be stable over a time of 0 to 60 minutes (Granot et al. 2003), it is possible that the repeated completion of VAS resulted in higher ratings. Because time alone did not affect pain tolerance and MPQ ratings, sensitization effects are less probable. Most notably, pain threshold was unchanged over the four conditions. It can be assumed that sensory threshold is strongly tied to the inherent properties of sensory receptors, and to intrinsic aspects of the pain experience. Results suggest that while pain threshold may not be separable from physiological aspects of pain perception, pain tolerance can be modulated by the cognitive and affective attitude, as for example, whilst empathizing with the identity of a *hero/heroine*.

The role of attention on the emotional components of pain perception has previously been demonstrated (Bantick et al., 2002; Villemure and Bushnell, 2002). Negative emotions can increase pain-directed attention (Rainville et al., 2005), and emotional salience of stimuli facilitates attention (Phelps, 2006). In addition, it has been shown that emotional vocal stimuli have a strong impact on brain dynamics, and attention magnifies this effect enabling emotion attention interactions to prioritize the processing of emotional events (Grandjean et al., 2005). It is still thinkable that the *hero* condition had a higher cognitive load capturing more attention. A pain stimulus would be then less of a distraction, resulting in higher tolerance values. Accordingly, it has been recently shown that a highly demanding task might distract attention from pain causing lower subjective intensity values (Veldhuijzen et al., 2006). Interestingly, we observed a significant *increase* and not a *decrease* of pain intensity ratings for *heroes/heroines*. Therefore, we strongly believe that the observed results were mainly influenced by emotional arousal induced by the emotional content -and not by differences in cognitive load of the story lines.

Anxiety-induced hyperalgesia has been reported (Rhudy and Meagher, 2000), whereas highly arousing negative affective states can attenuate pain (Janssen and Arntz, 1996). If anxiety were involved in the present results this fact would be congruent with the antithetic tolerance values of *heroes/heroines* and *faint-hearts*. On the other hand, if fear mediated the observed effects, attenuated instead of exacerbated pain perception would be expected during the *faint-heart* condition, something that was not observed.

*Heroes/heroines* attributed significantly more meaning to pain than *faint-hearts* did, and this correlated with more pain tolerance only of *heroes* and *heroines*, whereas *faint-hearts* showed less pain tolerance. Indeed, the *faint-heart* role was written free of passages containing tasks or motivations that would qualify pain as meaningful and suitable. Thus, pain was better tolerated as role identity conferred pain a meaningful and suitable character. Moreover, 58% of the freely named adjectives and phrases at the end of the *hero/heroine* role-playing story described emotions best fitting the role identity of a *hero* facing pain. Similarly, after the *faint-heart* condition, 89% of participants' descriptions were appropriate to a *faint-heart* facing pain. Furthermore, the terms *"hero/heroine"* or *"faint-heart"* were not explicitly mentioned at any time throughout the experiment. These data suggest that the used story lines induced the intended identities and associated emotions, which in turn may have altered pain perception.

It cannot completely be ruled out that listening to the *faint-heart* story may have lowered subjects' motivation to empathize with this role. Nevertheless, 89% of participants' descriptions were appropriate to a *faint-heart* facing pain, showing high empathy. Moreover, participants did not prefer one role to the other and SCL correlated during both role-playing stories. Thus, it appears unlikely that differences in motivation may explain the data. The actors and role players were experienced in empathizing with different roles and their level of role empathy was only about half of the intensity they would normally achieve during role-playing games. Therefore, to achieve a complete self-perceived role identity does not appear to be mandatory for a measurable change in pain perception. This fact might be of relevance in the eventuality that similar role inducing strategies are used for clinical purposes. Volunteers did not discern the real aim of the study, but the action of any induced role-identity could have continued into the heat testing phase, resulting in pain rating changes because of the actors continuing to act the role they empathized, the action of a role-identity trace or their conjoint action. This being the case, the implicitly given roles were able to modulate self-perceived role identity even after the story line or to transitorily induce emotional related states for periods longer than the role itself. All in all, such a scenario corresponds to the study aims.

The described effect of self-perceived role identity on pain sensation was gender unspecific. It might be argued that a higher number of participants will reverse these results. Nevertheless, such a sample-size effect would probably affect other calculations as well. Because overall, men showed higher pain tolerance than women, such an explanation is less likely. Therefore, data shows that women and men display equivalent emotional and cognitive skills confronted with the same painful situation. This is not surprising considering that, in modern times, gender roles are becoming increasingly similar. In keeping with this observation average skin conductance levels highly correlated for congruent female and male role identities (Figure 11). Most of the studies on acute and chronic pain showed that women are more sensitive to pain (Rollman et al. 2004). However, the effect size of these differences has been shown to heavily depend on method of pain induction and measurement, and on subjects' motivation (Riley et al., 1998). Results depict a different picture for pain tolerance compared to pain threshold. In agreement with Fillingim (Fillingim et al., 1998), data suggests that for induced heat pain, men have, overall, higher pain tolerance than women. Like others, no gender differences in pain threshold for induced heat pain were seen (Yosipovitch et al., 2004). Thus, different aspects of pain experience may lead to diverging results among genders, which warns against disproportionate generalizations.

This study does not allow for direct insights into action mechanisms. It is unlikely that results might have been influenced by hormonal status because the same persons experienced both roles. Moreover, circadian factors were controlled. On the other hand, future studies including analysis of cortisol levels may indicate to which extent role-induced functional modulation of the hypothalamic-pituitary-adrenal system was involved in the present results. In addition, neuroimaging studies may show whether empathizing with an archetype whatsoever, activates anterior insular-, and cingular regions of the brain, like during empathic pain, or whether specific forms of empathy, as for example role-empathy, are differently associated to more affective (Singer et al., 2004) or more sensory (Avenanti et al., 2005) patterns of brain activity. In addition, such studies may address the question as to whether during pain under a new role-induced identity, a global or a partial activation of the pain matrix occurs, and if dynamic changes in the activity of the endogenous opioid system can be observed (Apkarian et al., 2005; Sprenger et al., 2005).

## 5.5 Conclusion

This study demonstrated, that men and women are equally able to quickly and temporarily adopt two antithetic roles resulting in opposite effects on pain tolerance. This suggests an important role of self-perceived role identity, and its associated emotional status, on pain perception. It could be shown that the induced roles alleviated (*hero/heroine*) or aggravated (*faint-heart*) the emotional significance of noxious stimuli through alternative re-appraisal: increasing meaningfulness decreased their unpleasantness. Concomitantly, the action tendencies of participants changed. The *heroes/heroines* decided to endure the pain, while the faint-hearts suffered helplessly. Thus, the results of this study affirm, that an individual's behavioural response and attribution of emotional significance to a painful event is modified according to what is appropriate or possible in any particular situation. Modulating self-perceived role identity in emotionally meaningful settings may contribute to a beneficial influence on pain management. New treatments for pain conditions may benefit from exploring the use of similar imagery scenarios.

# 6

# Neurochemistry of Pleasure-related Analgesia

At first glance pain and pleasure appear to be both at the polar ends of the same scale. There is either pain *or* pleasure. To increase chances for survival we are primed to avoid the former and seek the latter (Leknes and Tracey, 2008). However, we often experience situations where both sensations are intertwined. Most often pain cuts pleasure down, but a certain amount of pain can also enhance pleasure, as for example when climbing a mountaintop, or eating spicy food. In a reverse relationship also positive emotional states have the power to shape pain perception. There is general agreement that pleasant emotional states reduce pain sensation, whereas unpleasant emotional states exacerbate it (see chap. 2.3.4). Yet the neural underpinnings of pleasure-related analgesia have hardly been explored and clearly deserve more attention. Recent studies in animals and humans have shown that an opioid-mediated descending pain modulatory system has the power to inhibit or facilitate pain. Particularly, the μ-opioid has been implicated in the regulation of both pain and emotional regulation (Ribeiro et al., 2005). However, until now studies have mostly explored the role of μ-opioid neurotransmission in both processes in isolation and not their interaction. The investigation of the role of endogenous opioid neurotransmission in the emotional modulation of pain, particularly in pleasure-related analgesia, was the aim of the following study.[14]

## 6.1  Objectives and hypotheses of the study

Pleasure-related analgesia, i.e. the phenomenon that pleasant emotional states alleviate pain, is of great interest for pain management therapies. However, the neural un-

---

[14] This study was published in March 2011 in *The Journal of Neuroscience* 31 (11): E. Kut, V. Candia, J. von Overbeck, D. Fink, G. Folkers: "Pleasure-related analgesia activates opioid-insensitive circuits".

derpinnings of this modulation are largely unknown and – surprisingly –hardly investigated. Since endogenous opioid neurotransmission has been shown to play a major role in the processing of pain and emotional states in a network of overlapping brain regions (see chap. 2.3.5), the starting point of this study was to assume that pleasure-related analgesia is at least partly mediated by this neurotransmitter system. It was hypothesized that during positive emotional states opioidergic neurotransmission is enhanced, which in turn leads to alleviated pain perception. The study investigated whether the reversal of μ-opioidergic activity by an injection of 0.2mg/kg naloxone, a predominantly μ-opioid-receptor antagonist, (a) attenuates the hedonic response to pleasant emotional stimuli (pictures) and (b) reduces pleasure-related analgesia. In specific, naloxone effects on following dependent variables were analyzed: heat pain tolerance, subjective pain intensity and unpleasantness (VAS), self-report on valence and arousal of experienced emotional state, autonomic reactions (eyeblink reflex magnitude and skin conductance level), and overall mood.

## 6.2  Design and methods of the study

Twenty-two healthy male volunteers (mean age 26.5, range 19–44) were included in the study. All participants had normal pain thresholds at the site of stimulus application, no history of neurological, psychiatric disease or drug abuse, no history of chronic or acute pain, and were not taking any form of analgesic, antidepressant, anti-anxiety or antihypertensive medication. Participants were asked to refrain from alcoholic beverages 12 h prior to the experiment. Handedness was determined using a standard handedness inventory (Chapman and Chapman, 1987). The study was conducted in accordance with the declaration of Helsinki on treatment of human subjects and was approved by the local research Ethics Committee and federal authorities. All participants gave written informed consent before participating in the study and were free to withdraw from the study at any time. They were instructed about the double-blind administration of naloxone and informed that no side effects were expected at the doses used. In addition, participants were told that the administered substance could increase, decrease, or, by no means at all influence pain perception.

At the beginning of each experimental session, participants were screened for medical problems (self-report) and given instructions on the procedure they were about to face. They all were told that the main aim of the study was on evaluation of the impact of emotional pictures upon the individual emotional state. In order to prevent participants from focusing on the used painful stimuli, and to focus their attention upon pleasure induction, the occurrence of noxious heat stimuli was mentioned, yet not as a principal study goal. After determining the weight of volunteers and after the insertion of the intravenous arm catheter, participants were seated in front of a monitor in a dimly lit room.

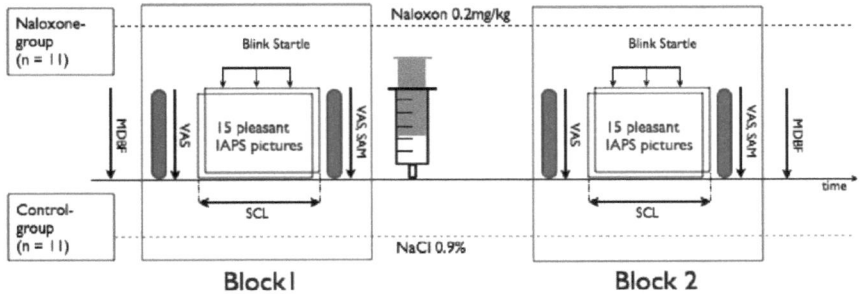

Figure 12: **Schematic depiction of an experimental session consisting of two blocks.** Each block (about 13 min. in length) included pain tolerance measurements before and after a period of picture viewing consisting of 15 pleasant IAPS pictures (180 seconds in total). Pain tolerance measurements were followed by subjective pain ratings. At the end of each block, subjective ratings on the emotional state during picture viewing were collected. In-between blocks, drug was administered followed by a 3 min distraction task. Red bars represent the use of noxious heat stimuli and their associated pain tolerance measurement. Vertical arrows represent scales and questionnaires displayed on a computer screen. Autonomic reactivity was measured during picture viewing periods during which three acoustic startle stimuli were presented (grouped vertical arrows). MDBF, Mehrdimensionaler Befindlichkeitsfragebogen; VAS, visual analogue scale; SAM, self-assessment manikin questionnaire; SCL, skin conductance level.

The experimenter affixed the thermode and the electrodes for autonomic reaction measurements and asked participants to follow the instructions presented via computer screen (SuperLab 4.0). The experiment was divided into two blocks preceded by a preparatory phase aimed at familiarizing participants with the experimental tasks (Figure 12). In each block one of the two picture sets was presented. Right before and after picture presentation pain tolerance succeeded by subjective pain ratings (VAS) were assessed. At the end of each block participants rated the affective state they had experienced while watching the pictures (SAM). Right before block 1, and immediately after block 2, mood ratings were assessed (MDBF). In-between blocks, naloxone or saline was administered. Special care was given, so that participants did not feel any pain or worry about the procedure. While waiting for the onset of naloxone effects after intravenous administration (approx. 2 minutes) and to distract subjects from the just experienced drug administration, a short (3 minutes) geometrical task was displayed on the monitor (meaningless geometric figure pairs had to be judged for similarity). The experiments were performed according to a randomized double-blind design in which neither the experimenter, the nurse, the medical doctor, nor the volunteers new which substance was administered. For security reasons (unforeseen side-effects of naloxone) the experimenter and the medical doctor stayed in the same room, behind a partition. To control for confounding factors associated to circadian variations, all participants were tested in the afternoon. At the end of an experimental session (total duration approximately 70 minutes) volunteers were debriefed about the experimental aims and received a monetary compensation for their participation in the study.

### 6.2.1 Data analysis

For pain tolerance measurements, subjective pain ratings and emotional ratings, repeated measurements ANOVA were performed. Within-subject factors were Block (block 1: before injection vs. block 2: after injection) and Time (before picture viewing vs. after picture viewing), with Group (naloxone vs. control) as between-subject factor. P-values in the ANOVAs and t-tests were corrected using Greenhouse-Geisser or Bonferroni correction, respectively. Post-hoc comparisons were performed using two-tailed Student's paired t-tests. Correlations between skin conductance levels and mean startle amplitudes were calculated separately for both groups using Pearson's correlation coefficient. In the analysis of subjective pain ratings, Grubb's test for outliers uncovered one outlier, which was therefore excluded from VAS-analyses. Significance level was set at $p<0.05$ for all statistical calculations.

## 6.3 Results

### 6.3.1 Expectation

17 of 22 participants, corresponding to 77% of the study sample believed they received saline. Two of the remaining participants thought they received naloxone and were indeed in the naloxone group while the remaining three were in the control group.

## 6.3.2 Pain tolerance

The repeated measurements ANOVA with the between-subject factor *Group* and the within-subject factors *Block* and *Time* was significant for the factor *Time* ($F_{1,20}$ = 29.61, p = 0.000), revealing that after picture viewing tolerances were higher. In addition, the factor *Block* was also significant meaning that in block 2 tolerances were lower ($F_{1,20}$ = 16.82, p = 0.001; Figure 13).

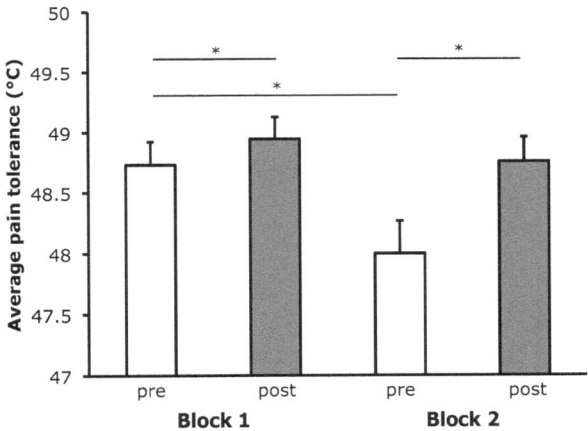

Figure 13: **Mean levels of heat pain tolerance (°C) pre- and post picture viewing in block 1 (before injection) and block 2 (after injection).** Pain tolerance increased significantly after picture viewing in both blocks and decreased after injection. Asteriks (*) indicate significant, post-hoc comparisons (P < 0.05). Bars depict average values and standard errors.

Moreover, the interaction *Block\*Time* was significant as well ($F_{1,20}$ = 18.54, p = 0.000). Post-hoc *t*-tests confirmed that pain tolerance increased significantly after picture viewing during both blocks (block 1: $t_{21}$ = -2.94, p = 0.008; block 2: $t_{21}$ = -5.67, p = 0.000), but decreased after injection (block 1 pre – block 2 pre: $t_{21}$ = 4.70, p = 0.000). The interaction *Block\*Group* and the interaction *Block\*Time\*Group* were not significant, suggesting that naloxone neither influenced pain tolerance, nor pleasure-related analgesia.

### 6.3.3 Subjective ratings of pain

For pain intensity, we found a significant main effect for the factor *Block* ($F_{1,19} = 5.35$, $p = 0.032$) uncovering that pain intensity ratings were higher after injection. Both scales showed a significant interaction *Block\*Group* (intensity: $F_{1,19} = 4.52$, $p = 0.047$; unpleasantness: $F_{1,19} = 4.31$, $p = 0.05$). Post-hoc t-tests uncovered that the naloxone group gave higher pain ratings after injection (intensity: $t_{10} = -3.48$, $p = 0.006$; unpleasantness: $t_{10} = -2.57$, $p = 0.028$) whereas the ratings of the control group did not change significantly (intensity: $t_9 = -0.12$, $p = 0.91$; unpleasantness: $t_9 = 0.12$, $p = 0.91$; Figure 14). The main effect *Time* or its interactions with the other factors were not significant.

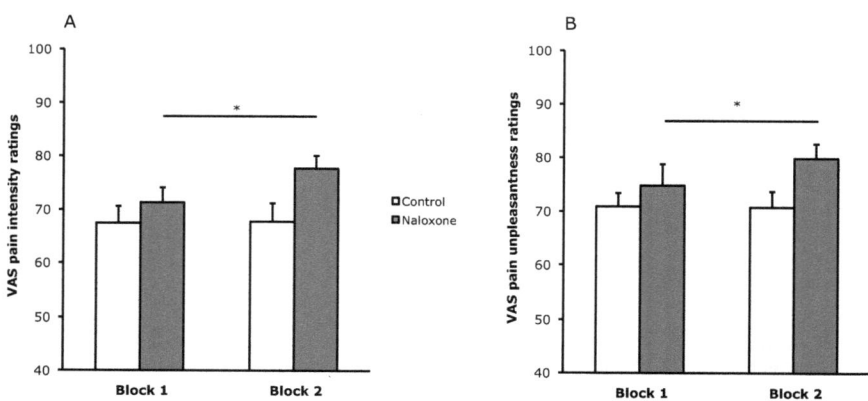

Figure 14: **Mean levels of subjective VAS ratings pre- and post picture viewing in block 1 and 2 for each group for (A) pain intensity and (B) unpleasantness.** In both groups subjective pain ratings did not significantly increase after picture viewing, although participants endured increased temperatures. Bars depict average values and standard errors.

### 6.3.4 Subjective ratings of emotion

Table 3 depicts subjective valence and arousal ratings for the emotional state of participants during picture viewing for blocks 1 and 2. These data confirm that indeed, the targeted pleasant emotional state was induced by the picture sets (mean valence > 7.1, mean arousal > 5.6).

Table 3: **Mean subjective ratings for the experienced emotional state during picture viewing (SAM valence and arousal) and mean mood ratings at the start and end of the experiment (MDBF).** The abbreviations for the dimensions of the MDBF questionnaire are: feeling well versus not well (w/nw), alert versus tired (a/t), and calm versus aroused (c/a). Values are means and standard error (S.E.).

|  | SAM valence | | SAM arousal | |
|---|---|---|---|---|
|  | Block 1 | Block 2 | Block 1 | Block 2 |
| Control (n=11) | 7.82 (0.23) | 7.00 (0.34) | 5.73 (0.20) | 6.09 (0.48) |
| Naloxone (n=11) | 7.27 (0.43) | 6.64 (0.53) | 5.45 (0.56) | 5.18 (0.56) |
| All (n=22) | 7.55 (0.24) | 6.82 (0.32) | 5.59 (0.29) | 5.64 (0.37) |

|  | MDBF (start) | | | MDBF (end) | | |
|---|---|---|---|---|---|---|
|  | w/nw | a/t | c/a | w/nw | a/t | c/a |
| Control (n=11) | 15.27 (0.94) | 13.82 (1.06) | 13.55 (1.32) | 14.00 (1.01) | 14.09 (1.36) | 13.64 (1.29) |
| Naloxone (n=11) | 15.55 (0.69) | 14.00 (0.78) | 14.55 (0.86) | 14.36 (1.09) | 11.64 (1.28) | 14.18 (1.03) |
| All (n=22) | 15.41 (0.57) | 13.91 (0.64) | 14.05 (0.78) | 14.18 (0.73) | 12.86 (0.95) | 13.91 (0.81) |

We found a main effect for the factor *Block* for SAM valence, but not so for arousal ratings (valence: $F_{1,20} = 6.43$, $p = 0.02$; arousal: $F_{1,20} = 0.03$, $p = 0.87$). The valence ratings for the emotional state decreased in block 2, yet they still mirrored highly pleasant states (mean > 6.8). We found no *Block\*Group* interaction for both scales, suggesting that naloxone did not alter hedonic responses to pleasant visual stimuli. Emotional state ratings for block 1 did not differ depending on picture set 1 (valence: 7.27 (S.E. = 0.42); arousal: 5.91 (S.E. = 0.34); n = 11) or picture set 2 (valence: 7.82 (S.E. = 0.23); arousal: 5.27 (S.E. = 0.47); n = 11), indicating that the emotional impact of both picture sets was equivalent (independent samples t-test for valence and arousal: $p > 0.27$).

## 6.3.5 Autonomic responses

Skin conductance levels (SCL) and startle magnitude during pleasure induction were analysed as autonomous markers of emotional state (Table 4).

Table 4: **Mean skin conductance level (SCL in µS) and startle eye blink magnitude (µV) as autonomous markers of emotional state during pleasure induction (i.e. 3min of picture viewing) across participants.** For every participant, SCL was averaged throughout picture viewing and startle eye blink magnitudes averaged across three startle probes presented during picture viewing per block. Values are means and standard error (S.E.).

|  | SCL | | Startle magnitude | |
| --- | --- | --- | --- | --- |
|  | Block 1 | Block 2 | Block 1 | Block 2 |
| Control (n=11) | 0.26 (0.03) | 0.24 (0.03) | 4.94 (0.91) | 4.95 (0.83) |
| Naloxone (n=11) | 0.31 (0.06) | 0.28 (0.04) | 5.42 (0.60) | 4.47 (0.79) |
| All (n=22) | 0.28 (0.34) | 0.26 (0.03) | 5.18 (0.53) | 4.71 (0.56) |

Averaged SCLs throughout the picture viewing periods were not significant for the main factor *Block*, nor the interaction *Block\*Group* (both p > 0.46). Conversely, correlation analyses between skin conductance levels in block 1 and block 2 were significant in both groups (control: rho = 0.47; p < 0.001; naloxone: rho = 0.48; p < 0.001), confirming that hedonic response in terms of SCL was not affected by naloxone. Analogously, averaged startle magnitudes during pleasure induction were not significantly altered by blockade of µ-opioidergic activity (*Block* and *Block\*Group*: p > 0.13).

### 6.3.6 Mood

Mood ratings (MDBF) at the beginning and the end of the experiment are depicted in Table 4. We found a main effect for the factor *Scale* ($F_{1,20}$ = 3.52, p = 0.05), whereby post-hoc t-test of scale ratings did not survive Bonferroni corrections, suggesting that ratings for *"feeling well versus not well"*, *"alert versus tired"* and *"calm versus aroused"* did not differ. Moreover, the interactions *Block\*Time* and *Block\*Group* were not significant (both p > 0.19), indicating that mood did not change in the course of the experiment and was not influenced by naloxone.

## 6.4 Discussion

The neural and chemical circuits underlying pleasure-related analgesia are not yet understood. However, the evidence that (a) positive emotional states are associated with high-level µ-opioidergic neurotransmission (Boecker et al., 2008; Leknes and Tracey, 2008) and that (b) µ-opioids attenuate pain, lead to a straightforward assumption. Pleasure-related analgesia, which is an increase in pain tolerance during positive emotional states, is mediated by activation of μ-opioidergic neurotransmission. This study investigated for the first time the effects of blocking opioidergic activity by naloxone, a predominantly μ-opioid-receptor antagonist, on emotional pain modulation. In specific, positive emotional states were induced through pleasant stimuli (IAPS pictures) and alterations of following dependent variables were measured: heat pain tolerance, subjective pain ratings, subjective and autonomic emotional response, and overall mood.

Positive affective states are associated with enhanced opioidergic activity (Boecker et al., 2008; Koepp et al., 2009) and negative states with its deactivation (Zubieta et al., 2003). Also the hedonic responses to external emotional stimuli such as sweet taste (Berridge, 2003), IAPS pictures (Gospic et al., 2008) and money reward (Petrovic et al., 2008) were shown to be modulated by opioids. In our study, mood and subjective ratings of experienced affective states during pleasant picture viewing were not significantly influenced by naloxone. Corroboratively, skin conductance responses, consistently shown to co-vary with arousal judgements (Lang et al., 1990), and the magnitudes of acoustically elicited startle eyeblinks, a reliable marker for the valence of an affective state (Lang et al., 1990), remained unchanged. Current hypotheses suggest that analgesia induced by viewing emotionally loaded pictures grounds on effects from changes in affective state and covariate, hardly dissociable attentional processes (Villemure and Bushnell, 2002). Since subjective and autonomic reactions to pleasure induction and overall mood neither differed between groups nor changed during the experiment, we suggest that the degree of attention was equivalent among participants.

Many studies have identified a major role of the endogenous opioid system in pain modulation by reversing its effects in the presence of naloxone (Gracely et al., 1983; Amanzio and Benedetti, 1999; Eippert et al., 2008) and using molecular imaging techniques (Zubieta et al., 2005; Scott et al., 2008). Our findings show that, pleasure-related analgesia, measured as an increase in pain tolerance, was insensitive to naloxone injection. After substance administration, we found a substance-unspecific decrease in pain tolerance. It is probable and even likely, that the procedure of drug administration (pressure in the vein) was responsible for these results. In line with previous findings on effects of naloxone on heat pain measurements, the increased level of subjective pain ratings of intensity and unpleasantness was substance specific (Borras et al., 2004). This result is highly appealing, as it suggests that μ-opioidergic neurotransmission is involved in the subjective response to heat pain. Because pain tolerances after pleasure induction were not attenuated by naloxone, it can be assumed that a major involvement of opioid-insensitive inhibitory systems is here at work. Studies on stress-induced analgesia and on placebo analgesia have similarly proposed the existence of opioid-sensitive and opioid-insensitive descending modulatory systems (Amanzio and Benedetti, 1999; Flor et al., 2002; Ford and Finn, 2008). Several neurotransmitter systems including dopaminergic, serotonergic, cannabinergic, and monoaminergic systems have been shown to play a role in endogenous pain inhibition but there still is a need for research on these systems (Millan, 2002). From a homeostatic perspective, the fact that reversal of endogenous μ-opioid neurotransmission did not significantly alter – at least at the behavioural level –hedonic processing and pain inhibition is comprehensible. The notion that both of them are maintained by different complementing, interacting and overlapping neural and chemical modulatory circuits, quickly equilibrating external disturbances, seems quite compelling if affective processes are conceptualized as action dispositions able to regulate and optimize an individual's response to motivationally relevant stimuli (Lang et al., 1990). Considering our limited sample size, our results should be cautiously interpreted. However, we are convinced that this study may provide indirect evidence for opioid-sensitive and, particularly, opioid-*insensitive* components of emotional regulation and modulation of pain experiences. Undoubtedly, the understanding of the neurobiological underpinnings of pleasure-related analgesia will be of great clinical benefit for the management of pain.

## 6.5 Conclusion

Both cognitive and emotional modulations of pain perception have been associated with a descending pain modulatory pathway that is, at least in part, mediated by endogenous opioids and reversible by naloxone. While the neurochemical underpinnings of cognitive effects on pain have frequently been investigated, as for instance in placebo and attentional studies, this study examined for the first time the contribution of endogenous opioids in emotional pain modulation. In contrast to placebo studies, where naloxone abolishes analgesia induced by expectation of pain relief, pleasure-related analgesia was robust to naloxone. Both hedonic response to pleasant visual stimuli and altered pain tolerances were not modified by μ-opioid receptor blockade. Strikingly, subjective pain intensity and unpleasantness ratings were sensitive to naloxone, suggesting that the appraisal of noxious heat stimuli is opioid-sensitive. These findings reveal that besides opioid-sensitive, particularly opioid-*insensitive* pain modulatory circuits are activated in pleasure-induced analgesia. The involvement and complex interactions of dopaminergic, serotonergic, cannabinergic and other neurochemical systems in emotional modulation of pain will need extensive research and may provide new target structures and mechanisms for the pharmacological and psychological treatment of pain.

# 7
# Synthesis and Outlook

The two main studies of this thesis (*role-identity* and *opioid study*) analyzed the effects of emotional state on pain perception using different approaches. While the *role-identity study* developed a tool to induce changes in self-perceived role identity leading to decreased pain perception in experimental or clinical settings, the opioid study investigated the neurochemical underpinnings of such emotional pain modulation. In the following an overall discussion, conclusion and outlook of this thesis will be given.

## 7.1 Synthesis

The overall discussion is divided in three chapters and various small sub-chapters in order to facilitate readability. However, delimitations between the chapters are by no means strict. I would like to add thoughts, concepts, and different views that chaperoned the realisation of this thesis. They emerged and developed during my time as a PhD student at the Collegium Helveticum, either in discussion with peers or in classic 'soliloquy' while writing, and would go beyond the scope of disciplinary scientific publications.

## I.

*The hurtfulness of pain*

A syllogism to start with: pain hurts.[15] Can the hurtfulness of pain be ascribed to a single feature when we consider the large variety of settings in which we find it in

---

[15] Many people would argue that this is a syllogism. Philosophical debates since the 18th century argue the hypothesis that pain only exists, when one feels it. Some say unfelt pains are like invisible rainbows, they can't exist, others disagree (Aydede, 2006, p. 59). Recent data suggests that pain is not exclusively a conscious event. A PET study in brain-damaged patients in a minimally conscious state indicates that they could have similar pain perception to healthy people, necessitating analgetic treatment of these patients (Boly et al., 2008).

common experience? Do we suffer from a sensory sensation, an emotion, or an aversion? Pain has typically all of the three dimensions, and others too. Pain can grab our attention in a distinctive way, oblige us to focus on a damaged tissue for example, and to mobilize resources to flee, fight or endure. Intense pain can disrupt all other thoughts or feelings. It can even temporarily affect our perception and appraisal of the world through altered visual, auditory and tactile sensations. These perceptual experiences again have emotional and motivational aspects to them that may be the result of the pain itself. It has thus been postulated, "pain is not the object of our perceptual experience, but rather, it is the experience itself" (Aydede, 2005). Pain encompasses the hurtfulness of the sensory sensation, the urgent desire that it ends, the anguish over the possibility that it will never end or even intensify, the disruption of thought and furthermore altered motivations and behavior. In line with this argumentation, current research in the sciences of pain point toward a conception of pain as an emotionlike, motivationlike, or needlike condition and not solely belonging to the category of sensations. Even more so, the new specific view of pain is of a homeostatic emotion, akin to temperature, itch, hunger and thirst (Craig, 2003).

## *Homeostasis*

> "La maladie est la plus respectée des médecines. A la bonté, au savoir, nous faisons des promesses, à la douleur, nous obéisons"
> – Marcel Proust

The bodies of all living beings are in constant dynamic activity. Hereby, several hierarchically organized homeostatic mechanisms maintain an optimal balance in the physiological condition of the body and guarantee for well being and survival against all environmental threats. Thus, pain keeps us alive, and what is more, in pain we feel alive. As a warning signal it urges us to avoid harmful situations and to take care of imminent or pathological processes, demanding action to diagnose and treat the underlying disease. However, in order to work efficiently to sign homeostasis disruption, the nociceptive system must be activated at a threshold sufficiently high to avoid impairment of normal functioning, but low enough to signal danger before it becomes effectively harmful (Ribeiro et al., 2005). Also the temporality of pain is a critical variable. Immediate response, but also termination of the pain experience is crucial for survival (see p. 83). When pain changes from acute to sustained or chronic the perceived emotional unpleasantness increases (Stohler and Kowalski, 1999). Frankly, one could say, we are at the mercy of pain throughout our lives.

## "I am in pain"

Nociceptive processing is based on physical and chemical events in the central nervous system and can hence be readily examined with objective methods. However, accessing the first-person experience of pain from an objective third-person perspective is a different kettle of fish (see chap. 2.2). In clinical situations, exactly this is the problem. Patients with certain forms of central nervous system damage or changes in neural structure may suffer from pain arising from an otherwise perfectly healthy body region, as for example seen in allodynia or neuralgia. Others may report no pain despite substantial tissue damage, as is often described in stressful situations as in a combat or an accident (see p. 83). Thus, a better understanding of both the pain experience and the development of methods for verbalising and communicating[16] pain have substantial practical importance.

To tackle the first-person experience of pain, subjective self-reports are used in clinic and research. It is interesting to note, that introspection, consists not only of 'inner observation' but also entails description and verbalization.[17] Since, unfortunately, most of us are barely poetically blessed, we face the problem that we cannot adequately describe a sensation such as pain or itch.[18] Our languages lack the proper words to describe a subjective state in such a way that someone who never experienced for example cluster headache or labor pain himself or herself, would get an idea of what that sensation is like, simply through the description.

Thus, how do we investigate this 'strange object of perception called pain' with scientific experimental tools? Especially, since besides the clinical urge to decipher pain mechanisms, pain can be regarded as a compelling model system for the study of how neural mechanisms support subjective experiences. The common way to tackle the pain experience, as also used in the presented studies of this work, is to assess first-

---

[16] In their current research Prof. Dr. Gerd Folkers and Nils Schaffner are developing and testing a new human-computer interaction device. It allows patients to express their perceived pain sensation in real time by using their intuitive bodily reactions to the acute pain.

[17] Further details on the introspection of emotional state on p. 129.

[18] Even those who *are* poetically blessed complain about the poorness of our languages to describe bodily sensations, as Virginia Woolf points at in "*On being ill*" ((Woolf, 1926/2002) "English, which can express the thoughts of Hamlet and the tragedy of Lear, has no words for the shiver and the headache. (…) but let a sufferer try to describe a pain in his head to a doctor and language at once runs dry. There is nothing ready made for him. He is forced to coin words himself, and, taking his pain in one hand, and a lump of pure sound in the other (as perhaps the people of Babel did in the beginning), so to crush them together that a brand new word in the end drops out." Notwithstanding, there are brilliant, consoling and at the same time and disturbing works portraying pain in music, art and literature, as for example "*Matthäuspassion*" of Johann Sebastian Bach and Fernando Pessoa's "*Livro do desassossego*" (Book of Disquiet). For a 'tour d'horizon' see (Hermann, 2006; Morris, 1994).

person subjective reports *and* third-person behavioural, psychophysical, and neurological measurements, such as EEG, PET, fMRI, in search of correlations among experiences, brain activity, and behavioural responses. I would like to emphasize that these correlations between conscious experiences and brain activity seem to map, irrespective of whether they are considered as two dimensions of one process or as two distinct things or properties connected in lawlike ways, as in the dualistic view.

## *On self-images*

"Cada um de nós é vários, é muitos, é uma prolixidade de si mesmos"
(Each one of us is several, is many, a profusion of selves/
Jeder von uns ist mehrere, ist viele, ist ein Übermass an Selbsten)
– Fernando Pessoa, Livro do desassossego, 1932

As open systems in a physical sense we are in steady exchange with the environment and obliged to continuously respond to signs and signals from the internal and external world that we are confronted with. We inherently appraise these inputs according to our belief and value systems, cultural background, past experiences, and emotional state and select from diverse interpretation alternatives. Motivations and action tendencies may change dependent on situation and self-conception. What is more, we are individuals in social systems naturally taking up positions and roles. Each role is accompanied by a set of expectancies of the environment and particularly of oneself that decisively influences behaviour in order to meet them. The painter Traversi once depicts a patient in a painful operation when forced and discouraged, with an agonising facial expression (Figure 6, above), and once calm and brave, close to a beautiful empathic woman (Figure 6, down). The perceived self-identity of the patient seems to influence the attribution of meaning to the tormenting event and changes its emotional impact, analogously to the *hero/heroine* in the *role-identity study*. It is an emotional rescaling of pain that takes place. Furthermore, the change of attitude appears to release inner resources to cope with the challenging situation.

In the publication of the results of the *role-identity study* we argued that the self-perceived role-identity (a) changes emotions and (b) the attribution of meaning to pain accordingly, which in turn affects intensity and quality of pain perception (Kut et al., 2007). I have the impression that the role identities used in the study have more facets than it was possible to discuss in the paper and would like to elaborate them here in detail.

## Meeting the role expectations

It can be presumed that the *hero/heroine* endeavours to tolerate intense pain, not only to save the princess, but also because the incentive to gain approval and leave a lasting impression is a very high reward. In this line of reasoning, a recent German study showed that the gender and professional status of the experimenter has a significant effect on the report and tolerance of pain in male and female healthy volunteers (Kallai et al., 2004). Subjects tolerated pain longer when they were tested by a professional experimenter and by an experimenter of the opposite sex. The latter indicates that it is not only men, as the authors expected, but also women who display increased pain tolerance when tested by a person of the opposite sex, most probably in order to impress this person. The authors assumed that women would follow the traditional gender role that was found in American samples (Levine and De Simone, 1991; Robinson and Wise, 2003) and show higher pain responsivity when tested by a male experimenter, in order to appear helpless and induce male protection. Cultural differences and the flux of gender roles at the present time may have lead to the heroic results of both male[19] and female students in this and accordingly in the *role-identity study*, where heroines were as brave as heroes.

The results indicate that pain responsivity, i.e. the will to endure pain as well as the report of pain, might be influenced in part by the characteristics of the person to whom the pain is expressed, which is a critical variable in clinical settings. During the experimental sessions of the *opioid study* we observed diverse behaviour of the confined male sample towards pain. Some volunteers endured the insertion of the needle and the painful heat stimuli without batting an eyelid, while others literally moaned behind the partition during pain tolerance measurements. In my impression, this groaning of some candidates was particularly expressed towards me, the female experimenter in the room, and scarcely towards the medical doctor, Jan von Overbeck. I am tempted to interpret this behaviour also as an attempt to impress as a hero, since Kallai et al. found that volunteers reported higher pain intensities when tested by female experimenters. In my opinion their interpretation that male participants might try to impress the female experimenters by saying that they were able to endure high pain intensities is quite reasonable. Or then again could it be, that these volun-

---

[19] In both the *psychophysics* and *role-identity study* two male participants had to be excluded from the data sets. All four of them exceeded the security limit of the heating device. Strikingly, in all cases a female experimenter carried out pain measurements.

teers – modern young men of a western society – tried to impress not by stoicism, but by their admitted sensitivity and openness to show their feelings?

## The status of employment as a substantive part of self-esteem

"According to the bundle theory of personal identity, there is no single and permanent self that persists through time; the self is rathera bundle of constantly changing and psychologicallycontinuous experiences or mental episodes."
– Evan Thompson, Mind in Life, 2007

It is a great fortune if one's research efforts are appreciated to be of value for the science and public community. We were very touched when we received an email by a patient[20] who was intrigued by the ideas and results of the *role-identity study*. Suffering for years from arachnoiditis, a neuropathic disease caused by the inflammation of one of the membranes that surround the nerves of the central nervous system, he wrote: "As a trained self observer I noted throughout that the pain was worse whenever my perceived status in society was lower i.e. I had less painful flare ups as a middle management supervisor than I had whilst working on the shop floor, but, paradoxically they were also lower when I was engaged in a capacity that allowed the 'hero' role to interject. By that I mean that whilst I was working a blue collar job that required physical input and dedication to the team ideal; where I was engaged in heavy lifting whilst running my own business, or, finally, when I was a coach and therefore role model for a group of young people. In all of these tasks it was easier to absorb the pain and keep going." These observations emphasize that individuals that find themselves in a position – and in western societies the status of employment is a substantive drive of self-esteem – that allows for high regard for themselves have stronger resources to cope with stressful events. "They are not heroes or heroines, just ordinary folk who have a strong personality, work ethic and positive frame of mind".[20] Thus, efforts have to be done, to develop – in addition to pharmaceutical pain treatment – strategies and regimes "aimed at raising the patient's own view of themselves and the world they now find themselves in". [20]

---

[20] Mike F. (United Kingdom), 20.8.2007

*Feelings of control*

The *hero/heroine* is in contrast to the *faint-heart* master of the situation. Although the role identity is embedded in an unavoidable, unpleasant context, he or she is prepared and eager to endure pain. Having a strong personality trait a *hero/heroine* perceives himself rsp. herself as able to cope with the painful situation, thus to be in conrol of it. As exemplified in chapter 2.3.2 clinical and experimental observations indicate that feelings of controllability are crucial for the management of acute and chronic pain. Perceived controllability attenuates the aversiveness of a noxious stimulus since the attribution of emotional significance diminishes its perceived menace. Similarly, anticipating, being anxious, and no longer having feelings of controllability about pain, as the *faint-heart*s did, can exacerbate the pain experienced.[21] Anticipating pain is highly adaptive, as for example everyone learns not to touch a hot stove. However, for the chronic pain patient it becomes maladaptive and can lead to fear of movement, avoidance, anxiety, and so forth.

The importance of controllability and anticipation is not restricted to pain, but to all life's challenges that we encounter in our daily life. Very interestingly, it was exactly these two dimensions, controllability and anticipation, that came up, when Jürgen Margraf replied to the question I raised during the recordings of Sternstunde Philosophie[22]: "What resources do we have in ourselves and in society to reinforce hope"? "Es gibt beim Bewältigen von negativen belastenden Erfahrungen, (…) zwei psychologische Dimensionen die extrem wichtig sind, und wenn wir die positiv beeinflussen, dann sind wir alle besser dran und das kann man: das ist die Vorhersagbarkeit und die Kontrollierbarkeit. Wir können sehr viel Stress aushalten, sehr viel Negatives aushalten, wenn wir es wenigstens vorhersagen können, noch besser, kontrollieren können. Wenn es uns also gelingt in unserer Erziehung und in unserer Gesellschaft den Menschen das Gefühl der Kontrolle und der Vorhersagbarkeit zu geben, dann geht es uns besser. Bei Kindern ist das bestens gezeigt. Man muss Kindern eine Möglichkeit geben, das Gefühl von Kontrolle zu entwickeln."

---

[21] Some researchers take this point to the extreme by advocating the occurrence of ‚psychogenic death' in situations of horror and utter helplessness. An overreacting emotional stress reaction may account for an acute drop in blood pressure and lead to heart failure.
[22] Sternstunde Philosophie (SF 1) in cooperation with Collegium Helveticum 10.4.2009: Angst und Hoffnung. Amrei Wittwer und Prof. Dr. Jürgen Margraf im Gespräch mit Dr. Norbert Bischofberger.

*The willingness to endure pain*

> "The art of true living in this world is more like a wrestler's, than a dancer's practice. For in this they both agree, to teach a man whatsoever falls upon him, that he may be ready for it, and that nothing may cast him down"
> – Marc Aurel, Mediations, seventh book[23]

There is a strong cognitive dimension in the role identity of a *hero/heroine* that we did not articulate in the paper: the willingness to endure pain. The change of emotional state that leads to an increase in pain tolerance was most probably induced intuitively when empathizing with the role. The willingness, however, to withstand the pain, doubtlessly also influenced the temperature the participants tolerated. I suppose that an increase of 2°C can be tolerated, if there is a willingness to do so. This mental attitude of the participant and also of a patient to his suffering is of high importance in pain therapy. The renowned poet Friedrich Schiller, trained as a physician himself, regarded pain, in a very modern sense, as a natural phenomenon caused by pathological events. In his lifetime he suffered from reoccurring agonizing attacks of pneumonia. It is known that he – at least *tried* – to overcome his pain through discipline and work. In his essay "*Über Anmuth und Würde*" (Schiller, 1793) he contemplates on the power of human will in shaping bodily conditions, such as pain: "Da einer Naturnothwendigkeit nichts abzudingen ist, so muß auch der Mensch, seiner Freiheit ungeachtet, empfinden, was die Natur ihn empfinden lassen will, und je nachdem die Empfindung Schmerz oder Lust ist, so muß bei ihm eben so unabänderlich Verabscheuung oder Begierde erfolgen. In diesem Punkte steht er dem Thiere vollkommen gleich, und der starkmüthigste Stoiker fühlt den Hunger eben so empfindlich und verabscheut ihn eben so lebhaft, als der Wurm zu seinen Füßen. Jetzt aber fängt der große Unterschied an. (…) Bei dem Menschen ist noch eine Instanz mehr, nämlich der Wille, der als ein übersinnliches Vermögen weder dem Gesetz der Natur, noch dem der Vernunft so unterworfen ist, daß ihm nicht vollkommen freie Wahl bliebe, sich entweder nach diesem oder nach jenem zu richten. Das Thier muß

---

[23] The German translation is even nicer: "Die Lebenskunst ist der Kunst des Ringens ähnlicher als der Tanzkunst, insofern nämlich, dass man gegenüber Schicksalsschlägen und Ereignissen, die man nicht hervorsehen kann, kampfbereit und fest dastehen muss."

sterben, den Schmerz los zu sein[24]; der Mensch kann sich entschließen, ihn zu behalten." Schiller continues, as if describing the painting of Traversi: "Da aber Züge der Ruhe unter die Züge des Schmerzens gemischt sind, (...) so beweist dieser Widerspruch der Züge das Dasein und den Einfluß einer Kraft, die von dem Leiden unabhängig und den Eindrücken überlegen ist, unter denen wir das Sinnliche erliegen sehen. Und auf diese Art nun wird die Ruhe im Leiden, als worin die Würde eigentlich besteht, obgleich nur mittelbar durch einen Vernunftschluß, Darstellung der Intelligenz im Menschen und Ausdruck seiner moralischen Freiheit." Tragically, it is also known that Schiller's pain attacks were often too excruciating than to be alleviated by willingness or idealism. His mental attitude together with *modern* pharmacological therapy would probably have given him considerable relief from his sufferings.

## *What neural circuits are involved?*

The neural mechanisms underlying the altered pain perception of a *hero/heroine* versus a *faint-heart* remain uncertain in the study. But, leaving aside the difficulties in understanding the enormously intricate circuits of the central neural system, how should one subsume the mental phenomena caused by role induction in order to investigate them? As elaborated above, a plethora of complex mental activities are induced when changing one's role-identity. There is for instance a change of appraisal of the situation. The threat of a negative event may contort. Changed self-awareness and perceived feelings of controllability may induce fear, anxiety or on the contrary courage, audacity and self-confidence. Very importantly, being able to attribute sense to a negative event may trigger the will to withstand it. Furthermore, we tend to fulfil expectancies or try to impress, for instance the doctor, the beautiful woman on Traversi's painting, or the tribe during a painful initiation ritual. Thus, to drink the potion of a *hero/heroine*, to put it metaphorically, entails diverse mental phenomena, such as expectation, attention, anticipation, positive and negative emotions, feelings of controllability, reappraisal and willingness – all variables that are usually investigated on their own to be specific and to reduce biases (see chap. 2.3).

---

[24] Evidently, Schiller wrote his essay in a time before Charles Darwin proposed a close relationship between the expression of emotions in animals and men (Darwin, 1872), and also before neurobiological research cemented that emotional and pain regulatory systems also in animals exist. Today, he would probably choose different comparisons to emphasize the power of the human mind.

II.

*The endeavour to design a follow-up study*

Growing evidence from placebo studies on pain strengthen the theory that mental processes, such as the mere thought and expectation of pain relief, influence neurobiological responses by leveraging neurotransmission and communication of neural circuits (Colloca and Benedetti, 2005). In other words, thoughts and expectations are able to trigger substrates in the body that have substantial effects on how we perceive, feel, or behave. Certainly, it is intriguing to speculate, that the way an individual perceives him-/or herself is associated with a set or level of neurobiological substrates and circuits. At first, it seemed promising to use an analogous experimental design as used in placebo studies[25] to investigate whether a neurotransmitter system as the endogenous opioid system is involved in role induced modulation of pain. The hypothesis would have been that role induction of a *hero/heroine* leads to an increase of opioid neurotransmission that in turn alleviates pain. Consequently, blockade of opioid neurotransmission with the μ-opioid receptor antagonist should – analogously to placebo studies – abolish role-induced analgesia. This idea seemed so plausible, that media took up the hypothesis and even graphically illustrated it during a short science programme in television on the *role-identity study*. But then again, having experienced at the point two years of critical discussion at the Collegium Helveticum, I had to heavily doubt the hypothesis. How could the injection of a single receptor antagonist block the feelings, beliefs, expectations and above all, the willingness of an individual to withstand pain? This would not only require that being a *hero/heroine* relies on a single neurotransmitter activity, but also that the paradigm of a single receptor-ligand interaction holds true. Apart from this categorical scepticism, there was another methodological unease. Even if the *heroes/heroines* of my future study would have exhibited altered μ-opioid neurotransmission, could I reveal it by measuring its blockade at the experiential level with pain tolerance measurements and subjective pain ratings?

These reserves made me focus on a specific aspect of self-awareness: the positive and negative set of emotions of a role-identity has and its influence on pain perception. Strangely enough, affective neuroscience has indulged for decades in the research of negative emotion and its effects on mental and physical health, as for example in

---

[25] In 1978 Levine et al. showed that placebo analgesia could be blocked by the opioid antagonist naloxone, which indicates an arbitrative involvement of endogenous opioids (Levine et al., 1978).

studies on fear, anxiety, helplessness, and catastrophizing (Edwards 06). Thus, instead of focusing on the emotional spectrum of a *faint-heart* and its pain exacerbating consequences, the positive emotions of a *hero/heroine* that contribute to an increased pain tolerance aroused my interest. I turned to the question: what are the biological correlates of the beneficial effects of positive emotional states, such as pleasure on pain perception?

## *Pain and pleasure*

> "Alles geben die Götter, die unendlichen,
> ihren Lieblingen ganz,
> alle Freuden, die unendlichen,
> alle Schmerzen, die unendlichen, ganz."
> – Johann Wolfgang von Goethe

Pronounce the words pain and pleasure and listen. Don't they make you feel different? There is suppleness in the word pleasure, smooth, warm, relaxing, even voluptuous. Every syllable seems to melt in the mouth. Pain – a short, spiky, sharp word, like a gunshot. We have an innate affinity to seek pleasure and to avoid pain and whatever we do, whichever decision we make, is at the bottom formed by the competitive interaction of these strong motivators. Shall one pick the forbidden fruit to cherish its sweetness to the cost of burning one's fingers?

"Sometimes there's so much beauty in the world I feel like I can't take it, like my heart's going to cave in" are the words from the movie *"American Beauty"*[26] that describe the sensitivity an individual feels when pleasure becomes almost painful. Buddhists consider life as constant suffering, because we are condemned to loose, whatever we love. Precious moments go by, beloved persons leave us, stocks loose their value, and feelings fade away. But isn't it precisely the tension, the contrast of pain and pleasure that flavours each sensation, as Jaak Panksepp puts it: "Our capacity to love is built partly upon our ability to experience loss" (Panksepp, 2005). It appears, that pain and pleasure are binary elements that form – ideally – a balanced unity. Personally, I cherish also the bittersweet tastes in life.

---

[26] American Beauty, directed by Sam Mendes, USA, 1999.

The pain–pleasure dilemma has a long tradition in the history of humanity.[27] The stoic doctrine of temperateness towards pain and pleasure has had a lasting influence on western cultures. In combination with the Christian notion of shame and moderation the unregulated seeking for pleasure is utterly beyond social conventions. Nowadays, the call for moderation is supported by neuroscientific research. Prominent addiction researchers emphasize that the use of the reward system should be restricted, as they believe that unregulated pleasure-seeking might lead to it's dysregulation and result in addiction (Koob and Le Moal, 1997).

Thus, the hedonic experience of pain and pleasure is strongly biased by our cultural background and moral norms and obviously, not only by inherent homeostatic drive of avoiding pain and seeking pleasure. The religious ascetic or masochist welcomes pain, though for different motives. Pain can trigger pleasure. When wasabi diffuses up our nose as if reaching the brain, when we scratch a mosquito bite, until it eventually starts bleeding, or when we bathe in a incredibly hot spring, we may simultaneously shiver with pleasure. And what is it that constantly makes us touch a limb, scab or mental wound to check whether it still hurts? Some say, in pain we feel alive.[28]

*Pleasure-related analgesia*

Experimental studies have investigated scenarios were pain and pleasure are superimposed. Undoubtedly, being in pain cuts back pleasure. There are a few ambivalent situations, when pain enhances pleasure (see above). However, also pleasure modulates pain by decreasing it. This phenomenon, called pleasure-related analgesia, has been reported in studies measuring experimental pain after exposing participants to pleasant picture, films, and other pleasure-inducing stimuli (see 2.3.4). Pleasure-related analgesia originating from sexual action has until now – at least to my knowledge – only been systematically tested in mice, probably for the obvious ethical obstacles in carrying out these kind of studies (Leknes and Tracey, 2008). Astonish-

---

[27] See for example Leonardo da Vinci's drawing *Allegory of pleasure and pain*. "This represents pleasure together with pain, and show them as twins because one is never apart from the other. They are back to back because they are opposed to each other; and they exist as contraries in the same body inasmuch as the origin of pleasure is labour and pain, and the various forms of evil pleasure are the origin of pain." (Notebooks of Leonardo da Vinci, Volume 1, chapter X, translated by J. P. Richter 1880).

[28] "I hurt myself today, to see if I still feel, I focus on the pain, the only thing that's real". The Lyrics of the song *"Hurt"* by the music band Nine Inch Nails describe the experiences patients may have that suffer from borderline personality disorder and depressive disorders, often deliberately hurting themselves to overcome numbness or relieve otherwise unbearable emotions.

ingly, these aforementioned human studies have only investigated the experiential aspects, but did not approach the neural underpinnings of the emotional modulation of pain that is largely unknown and of possible insight for pain management strategies.

There are two main theories on mechanisms of emotional modulation of pain that researchers mostly refer to. In my opinion, they are quite similar although most authors refer to either one or the other. According to the 'Motivational Priming Theory' emotions are driven by two opponent primary motive systems. These are an appetitive system, associated with positive affect, responding to for instance nurturant or sexual cues and engendering approach behaviours, and an aversive system, associated with negative affect, responding to threat and promoting avoidance behaviours (Lang, 1995). Lang and co-workers studied extensively the startle reflex that was also used in the *opioid study* (see chap. 6 ), to show how pleasant emotional states attenuate the defensive system: pleasant pictures reduce the startle magnitude (Lang et al., 1990). The same neural circuit that mediates emotional modulation of the startle reflex has been implicated in pain modulation. Thus, according to the Motivational Priming Theory exposure to pleasant images inhibits pain by activating the appetitive system. The 'Motivation-Decision Model' of Fields also bases on the premise that emotions emerge as a result of knowledge on impending threats or available rewards together with information about the homeostatic state of the individual, and the quality of sensory input (Fields, 2007). In a conflicting situation, thus when there is something potentially more important for survival than pain, as for instance hunger or a threatening predator, or the reward is just so very seductive, pain is suppressed. These antinociceptive effects allow attention to focus to the more important event.

## *Pain: imprinting and being imprinted*

In the introduction of this work I outlined that pain is a potent motivational drive that can thoroughly dominate attention. As a guardian of survival pain urges us to refrain from potential harm. Obeying to the warning signal we avoid threats for the body and 'the soul', as for example in the case of social exclusion pain (see p. 95). Considering the abovementioned theories of Lang and Fields I come to realize that pain has a duality that I haven't elaborated yet. Pain can either be a motivational drive itself, or subject to more important motivational states, such as the aversive and appetitive systems. The decision on how to respond to a threat is the outcome of a weighting between the urgency of a threat or reward and the pain, from for example an ongoing tissue-damage (Fields, 2004). In a manner of speaking, the cost-benefit ratio determines the reaction. It is a known phenomenon that wounded people on a battlefield or after an accident transitorily may not feel their injuries (Melzack et al., 1982). Hence, pain is a dynamic sensation that shapes subsequent behaviour, and is being shaped by it. It is at the same time commander and subordinate. In other words, the neural circuits of pain processing simultaneously contribute to behaviour and decision-making and are in a reverse relationship determined by it.

## *Activation of opioid circuits*

The preceding paragraph postulates a biological imperative for pain modulation. Successive animal and human studies have given evidence that nature provided us with an opioid-sensitive pain-modulatory pathway to get through painful situation (see chap. 2.2.2). This pain relieving circuit includes prefrontal, anterior cingulate and insular cortices, amygdala, hypothalamus and brainstem structures like the periaqueductal grey, and the descending projections to the spinal dorsal horn. Most interestingly, it can not only inhibit, but also facilitate nociceptive input. Its activation has been shown in mice during both appetitive and aversive motivational states (Fields, 2004). The appetitive cues were hereby feeding of sucrose, and the aversive cues, the presence of an aggressive male conspecific or inescapable foot shock.

Various evidences suggest that opioids can be regarded as a chemical interface between pain and emotion (Bodnar, 2008). Opioids such as morphine and heroin produce aside from powerful analgesia "profound appetitive motivational actions" (Fields, 2004) or – in plain terms – feelings of euphoria.[29] Comprehensive research in mice (Boecker et al., 2008; Burgdorf and Panksepp, 2006; Fields, 2007; Panksepp, 2003; Zubieta et al., 2003), and PET ligand-activation studies in humans (Boecker et al., 2008; Zubieta et al., 2003) have shown that endogenous µ-opioid neurotransmission mediates the regulation of emotional states, as for example in the hedonic response to pleasant stimuli (Berridge, 2003; Pecina, 2008) (see chap. 2.3.5). The num-

---

[29] First records from Sumerians (approximately 3000 B.C.) refer to the poppy plant as 'Hul Gil', the plant of joy (Brownstein, 1993). The use of Opium as a medicine for *body and mind* throughout history is tremendously fascinating. It spans from the cultivation of Papaver somniferum in lower Mesopotamia (3000 B.C.), famous potions of physicians such as Galen (2nd century A.D.) and Paracelsus (16th century), to opium wars in China (19th century), and to pharmacological extraction of morphine (1803) and synthesis of heroin (1874). Many famous people, such as Marc Aurel, Charles Baudelaire, John Keats, and Friedrich Glauser, and countless more nameless people have tasted its highest heights and lowest depths. The widely known addictive properties of opioids receive widespread interest in addiction research.

ber of references suggesting that both painful and pleasant emotional states are associated with high-level μ-opioidergic neurotransmission eventually led to the conception of the *opioid study*. It was hypothesized that the enhanced μ-opioidergic neurotransmission during positive emotional states contributes to pleasure-related analgesia. The main result of the opioid study was that pleasant emotional states and pleasure-related analgesia was also induced after completely blocking μ-opioidergic neurotransmission. Naloxone however increased subjective ratings of pain intensity and pain unpleasantness. These results indicated that regulation of both pain and hedonic response to pleasant stimuli – at least at behavioural level – are not solely dependent on the release of endogenous opioids and other regulating systems of affect and pain were predominantly activated. In the following I would like to give an in-depth discussion on the results, caveats of interpretation and implications for the field of emotional pain research.

## *Placebo, naloxone and the pain-modulatory system*

Fields postulated that the activation of opioid-mediated pain-modulatory circuits is driven primarily by motivational state (see p. 82). There is significant support for this hypothesis coming from the investigation of psychosocial analgesic effects in humans: the placebo response. In terms of motivational processes the expectancy and desire for pain relief is a rewarding cue assigning placebo analgesics appetitive motivational power. Therefore, it can be expected that a person anticipating and desiring pain relief engages his or her opioid-mediated circuit. The involvement of the endogenous opioid system in placebo analgesia was first suggested in 1978, when it was shown that an opioid receptor antagonist (naloxone!) was able to block placebo-induced analgesic effects (Levine et al., 1978). These first observations where then corroborated across multitudes of psychophysical and imaging studies highlighting the involvement of opioid-mediated descending pain modulatory circuits (Amanzio and Benedetti, 1999; Petrovic et al., 2002; Zubieta and Stohler, 2009). A particularly interesting study showed that the same brain regions are activated by both a placebo and the opioid agonist remifentanil, indicating analogous mechanisms underlying mentally and pharmacodynamically induced analgesia (Petrovic et al., 2002).

## Naloxone-sensitive and –insensitive inhibitory pathways

Although the role of endogenous opioids in cognitive pain modulation, such as placebo analgesia, is widely acknowledged and ever so often quoted, the state of affairs is – not surprisingly – more complicated. Already in 1983 the existence of time-dependent, non-opioid components of placebo analgesia, i.e. that are not reversible by naloxone, were postulated (Gracely et al., 1983; Grevert et al., 1983). Since then, the activation of opioid and non-opioid systems in placebo analgesia has been tackled several times. Since the outcomes might be of insight for the interpretation of the naloxone-insensitive analgesic effects in the *opioid study*, I would like to exemplify some data from placebo research. It appears that opioid and non-opioid mechanisms come into play under different circumstances (Colloca and Benedetti, 2005; Fields and Levine, 1984). Thus, when investigating activations of naloxone-reversible and naloxone-insensitive placebo responses, the procedure of placebo treatment, as for example verbal suggestion or drug conditioning with an opioid such as morphine, has to be taken into account. In a model of experimental ischemic arm pain for example, the placebo response was blocked by naloxone, when it was induced by strong expectation cues (Amanzio and Benedetti, 1999). Reduced expectation cues lead to a placebo response that was insensitive to naloxone.[30] Moreover, it appears that while strong expectation triggers endogenous opioids, conditioning activates specific subsystems (Amanzio and Benedetti, 1999). Most authors avoid speculating on the neurobiological nature of possible specific subsystems, in other words on naloxone-insensitive inhibitory systems. This is probably due to the fact that most experimental paradigms, including the *opioid study*, do not allow the identification of the mechanisms of these other systems.

## Non-opioid mechanisms

A multitude of transmitters and mediators is involved in the transmission and modulation of nociceptive processing in the dorsal horn and higher brain areas. An "inventory" of these players extends in 120 pages and is mind-blowingly complicated (Millan, 2002). Besides endogenous opioid systems there are cannabinoid, serotonin, do-

---

[30] For related thoughts on the intensity of emotion induction in the *opioid study* see p. 130.

pamine, glycin, GABA[31], histamin, adenosine and cholinergic systems, and many others. An in-depth discussion of these systems that most probably played a major role in pleasure-related analgesia in the *opioid study* would go beyond the scope of this thesis. Still, I would like to highlight some research in this field that I find quite compelling.

Besides endogenous opioids, dopamine is a prime candidate for mediating the mutually inhibitory effects of pain and positive emotional states. There is robust evidence for the involvement of dopaminergic pathways in pain and reward processing coming from animal and human studies (Magnusson and Fisher, 2000). In placebo analgesia for instance, the activation of both neurotransmitter systems was found in the nucleus accumbens, a core area in neural reward circuitry (Scott et al., 2007, 2008). Using [$^{11}$C]raclopride, a D2-D3 dopamine receptor agonist, and [$^{11}$C]carfentanil, a μ-opioid receptor agonist, and fMRI, they were able to show a significant correlation between the responsiveness to placebo and that to monetary reward. Opioid and dopamine systems interact in very complex ways, up- and downregulating each other depending on their phasic or tonic levels and involved brain areas (Leknes and Tracey, 2008). If we consider the Motivation-Decision Model that suggests that temporary inhibition of pain in order to gain a reward could increase survival, if the pain-pleasure ratio – or in other terms the 'cost-benefit' ratio (p. 83) – is right, the interplay of opioid and dopamine systems is evident (Fields, 2004; Fields, 2007). Both neurotransmitters may be regarded as brain's common currency for pain and pleasure, processing both pleasant and aversive information and mediating action tendencies. An intriguing fMRI study demonstrated that noxious thermal stimuli of 46°C produce significant activation in classic pain circuitry as well as in putative reward circuitry (Becerra et al., 2001). Most interestingly, in the nucleus accumbens the direction of the signal change appeared to be opposite for aversive versus rewarding stimuli. This not only lends support to the view that pain and pleasure are at the opposite ends of the same behavioural spectrum (see p. 81) but also introduces a means by which emotional stimuli could quickly modulate pain perception.

---

[31] During the 5 years research period on emotions at the Collegium Helveticum (2004–2009) fellow Hanns Möhler was involved in a study investigating the contribution of benzodiazepine receptor subtypes in chronic pain states in mice (Knabl et al., 2008; Zeilhofer et al., 2009). The pioneering results, published in Nature 2008, show that targeting a specific subset of GABA$_A$ receptors provide pronounced antihyperalgesic activity against inflammatory and neuropathic pain. These results provide a rational basis for the development of subtype-selective GABAergic drugs for the treatment of chronic pain, devoid of the typical side-effects of classical benzodiazepines.

*Receptor affinities and pharmacological antagonisation*

As introduced in chapter 2.2.3 the endogenous opioid system consists of three major opioid receptor classes: μ, δ, κ, and further opioid-like (orphan) receptors and probably other undiscovered ones. They are characterised by different distribution, discrete affinities towards multiple endogenous ligands, and broad functional diversity. Binding assays in homogenates of animal brain tissue – mostly male rats are thereto "sacrificed by cervical dislocation"–, and the use of newly cloned rat and human opioid receptors allow for the characterisation of their pharmacological profile and structure-function analysis (see below).

The κ-receptor exhibits the greatest degree of selectivity across endogenous ligands with affinities ranging from 0.1 nM for dynorphin to approx. 100 nM for Leu-enkephalin – i.e. a 1000-fold range. In contrast, μ- and δ-receptors only have a 10-fold difference between the most- and least-preferred ligand. The relatively unimpressive affinity of the μ-receptor towards all known endogenous ligands led to the discovery of its yet most avid and selective ligands: endomorphin-1 and endomorphin-2 (Zadina et al., 1997). These partial agonists show a remarkable affinity and selectivity for the μ-receptor (Horvath, 2000). At the time Levine et al. showed in 1984 that the μ-opioid antagonist naloxone only partially inhibits placebo response and thus advocated opioid and non-opioid mediated pathways, only the existence of β-endorphins as a natural ligand of μ-receptors was known. Astonishingly, authors in placebo research advocate the same argumentations, not mentioning novel and broadened knowledge on the endogenous opioid system, and the discovery of endomorphins in particular.

Because of the widespread reliance upon naloxone to define μ-opioid systems, the interpretations of these experiments should be tempered by certain pharmacological considerations. When talking about ligand-receptor activities as occurring in blockade of neurotransmitter systems one has to consider receptor and ligand properties. Ligand binding is often characterized in terms of the concentration of ligand in mol per litre at which half of the receptor binding sites are occupied, known as the equilibrium dissociation constant $K_d$.[32] If the $K_i$ is low, the affinity of the receptor for the

---

[32] In competitive binding studies usually the term $K_i$ for binding affinity is used. $K_i$ values are determined using a competitive binding assay, i.e. an assay based on the competition between a radiolabelled ligand, such as [$^3$H]-DAMGO and an unlabelled ligand, as for example morphine, in the reaction with a receptor. DAMGO [D-Ala$^2$,N-Me-Phe$^4$,Gly-ol]-enkephalin is a highly selective ligand for μ-opioid receptors and often used in binding assays.

ligand is high. Differences in the experimental conditions, that is, the materials studied, the membrane preparation protocols, or the choice of radioactive ligands lead to varying $K_i$ values. The online $K_i$ database of the National Institute of Mental Health's Psychoactive Drug Screening Program[33] lists an overview of published binding properties of a great number of G-protein coupled receptors, ion channels, transporters and enzymes. The range of reported binding affinities of β-endorphin, endomorphin-1, endomorphin-2, naloxone, and morphine are listed in Table 5.

Table 5: **The range of published binding affinities ($K_i$) of different ligands at the μ-receptor.** The results are retrieved from the online $K_i$ database PDSP gathering published data from receptor binding assays using cloned animal and human μ-receptors or animal brain homogenates respectively; each range comprises the results of 6 – 8 independent publications.

|  | μ-receptor |
|---|---|
| β-Endorphin | 0.94–2.3 nM |
| Endomorphin-1 | 0.24–5.3 nM |
| Endomorphin-2 | 0.43–6.9 nM |
| Naloxone | 0.56–1.5 nM |
| Morphine | 1.0–6.6 nM |

The binding affinities listed in Table 5 have quite a range. Does naloxone then really block *all* endogenous opioid binding at the μ-receptor? This is a crucial question, since it is often advocated that naloxone-insensitive components of pain inhibition have to be genuinely non-opioid mediated.

If we assume a $K_i$ for naloxone of 0.56 nM and a $K_i$ of 0.24 nM and 0.43 nM for endomorphin-1 and endomorphin-2 respectively, than the endomorphins bind stronger to the μ-receptor than naloxone. In other words, naloxone will not be able to competitively displace the endogenous ligands. However, and this is striking, in vivo animal studies demonstrated dose-dependent analgesia of endomorphins on different nociceptive methods that were all *reversed* by naloxone (Horvath, 2000; Li et al., 2001). In accordance with these findings, a multitude of other animal studies, mostly in rats,

---

[33] NIMH PDSP: http://pdsp.med.unc.edu/pdsp.php (2009).

showed that naloxone is also able to significantly antagonize antidepressant-like, cardiovascular, respiratory, sexual, cholinergic and other effects of endomorphins (Fichna et al., 2007). Autoradiographic studies in rat brain membranes also strongly support the view that naloxone blocks endomorphin binding to µ-opioid receptors (Goldberg et al., 1998). These novel evidences and previous research (Hill, 1981) robustly suggest that naloxone antagonizes *both* β-endorphin and endomorphins at the µ-opioid receptor. Thus, when interpreting the results of the *opioid study* and other studies using naloxone antagonisation, such as placebo studies, one might reasonably identify naloxone-insensitive mechanisms as non-opioid mediated mechanism, or at least not µ-opioid mediated.

δ- and κ-opioid neurotransmission can also excert antinociceptive, or in the case of κ, pronociceptive effects (Millan, 2002). It could be assumed that blockade of µ-opioid receptors in the *opioid study* was compensated by antinociceptive effects of the other opioid receptor classes, which is known as 'cross-talk' interaction. However, studies in µ-opioid receptor knockout mice have failed to detect compensatory changes in either the localization or signal transduction of δ- and κ-receptors (Matthes et al., 1998). Nevertheless, since naloxone probably blocked only a part of δ- and κ-receptors due to low affinity[34], antinociceptive contributions of these receptors to pleasure-related analgesia cannot be ruled out.

## *Women and men*

From the perspective of a pharmacologist women are an incredibly strange entity to study. They have hormonal cycles stirring up metabolic and emotional parameters. What is 'worse' they can get pregnant thereby answering for the health of the offspring via placenta or breast-milk. Thus, it is better to beware of female volunteers – that is at least what Swissmedic advised us to do. The *opioid study*, though planned and permitted by the cantonal ethical committee for both gender, was finally carried out only in men, complying with the constraints of the federal authorities.[35] The irony of the research venture wanted it that the experiments were carried out in collaboration with the gynaecologists Daniel Fink and Judit Pók in the rooms of the department of gynaecology at the University Hospital Zurich. At least, this fact simplified

---

[34] The $K_i$ of naloxone for δ is 17 nM and 2.3 nM for κ respectively (Raynor et al., 1994).
[35] On a side mark: The application for approval of the *opioid study* lasted for 16 months, since federal and cantonal authorities adhere to regulations that are strangely feed-back looped.

the spotting of male volunteers in the hallway. Though the results of the *opioid study* therefore do not provide insights on gender differences in naloxone-sensitivity of pleasure-related analgesia, I would like to mention some interesting findings from literature. There is an ongoing debate on gender differences in pain perception. In experimental pain studies men tolerate more pain than women, as also seen in the *psychophysics* and *role-play studies* (see chap. 4.3.2 and chap. 5.3.1). Some authors call on estrogen level, or athletic state, others rather on socio-cultural factors, such as the role expectation of the woman as 'the weak sex' (Fillingim et al., 2005; Robinson et al., 2003). Growing evidence suggests that there are substantial gender differences in endogenous opioid systems (Ribeiro et al., 2005). Dynamic ligand-PET studies demonstrated that at identical pain magnitude men exhibit greater μ-opioidergic activation in pain processing areas than women (Sprenger et al., 2005; Zubieta et al., 2002). What is more, women may even respond with deactivation of endogenous opioid neurotransmission to sustained pain and sadness, associated with increased ratings of negative affect and pronounced pain unpleasantness (Zubieta et al., 2003; Zubieta et al., 2002). In this regard, a bidirectional role of this neurotransmitter system in the generation or maintenance of pain and emotional states has been suggested and may partly account for marked behavioral variability observed in pain, stress and emotional responses (Ribeiro et al., 2005; Smith et al., 2006). These findings intriguingly show, that we can only gain comprehensive understanding of human 'functioning' by investigating both males and females.

## III.

### *"Reflection kills desire"*

Emotion research cannot do without taking the first-person perspective into account. Subjective ratings and qualitative interviews are common means to systematically approach the subjective dimension – or qualia – of emotions or pain. However, these inquiries entail pitfalls and can introduce confounding effects. For example, one might ask, to what extent introspection changes the experience of pain or any experience. Or, even more interesting, to what extent does the pain or emotion that one tries to introspect actually affect the introspection? It has been postulated that 'reflection kills desire'. Some researchers ask their participants to give ratings on the experienced emotions *during* picture viewing periods, in order to accurately check emotion induction (de Wied and Verbaten, 2001). Imagine immersing yourself in a picture set of 15 pleasant pictures – and having to rate each single one of them right afterwards. How much pleasure can thereby arise? In the *opioid study* I therefore decided, to minimize inquiry to one rating for the whole picture set *after* picture viewing for the benefit of actual pleasure induction. There are interesting findings on neural processes underlying verbalizing of negative emotions. We have a long tradition of talking about sorrow: A sorrow shared, is a sorrow halved. This has been formally practiced for more than a century in talk therapies. Recent fMRI studies have now shown that affect labelling, which simply means putting feelings into word, may diminish the impact of negative emotional events on current experience along a pathway from prefrontal cortex areas to the amygdala (Lieberman et al., 2007). The results indicated that affect labelling diminished the response of the amygdala and other emotion-related regions to negative emotional pictures. In a way, these findings give a preliminary answer to the first question raised above, indicating that the act of verbalizing an emotion already shapes its experience.

*Emotion induction*

It should not be too difficult to induce feelings of stress or anxiety in experimental paradigms. A study participant most often already feels disconcertingly scrutinized and tends to maintain these feelings during the whole experiment. Distinct personality traits and individual mood of subjects in a certain study sample may lead to confounding effects and complicate all studies with human beings, particularly in affective neuroscience. The challenge I was facing, was how to shift participant's perceived self-identity in the direction of a *hero/heroine* (*role-play study*), or even induce highly pleasant emotional states (*opiod study*). For the former, we decided to use self-written role-plays that were inspired by a famous fantasy role-playing game. We soon realized that the voice of the speaker has fundamental consequences on the power of role induction and therefore on the success of the study. The sound waves of a voice communicate emotions. When Gerd Folkers, with his sonorous and thus suitable reader voice, performed the role-plays, there was a subtle irony imbedded in the sound. We feared, that this irony might hinder participants from thoroughly immersing themselves in the fantasy stories. The best solution we then found was to have a professional speaker reading the role-plays, who was trained to control and accurately bring in emotions. Fortunately, the results confirmed the effectiveness of the professionally performed role-plays in inducing the *hero/heroine* or *faint-heart* role (see chap. 5.3.4).

For the *opioid-study* I had to select an emotion induction method that is effective in inducing highly pleasant emotional states involving opioid release. At the same time the emotional stimuli were required to be standardised and established in the research community in order to guarantee for comparability and reproducibility of the findings and convince reviewing boards. The International Affective Picture System (IAPS) is a milestone of emotion research. It consists of over 600 colour pictures from magazines, newspapers and books. The emotional impact of the *pleasant* pictures, showing families, romantic or erotic love, food, and sports, the *unpleasant* pictures, depicting violated corpses, mutilations, disgusting sceneries, and guns, and the *neutral* pictures of household objects, plants, and landscapes, have been rated along the valence and arousal scales by hundreds of volunteers in various studies (Lang et al., 2004). Although viewing slides is a relatively subtle manipulation, physiological reactivity, as measured in changes of skin conductance, heart rate, and startle magnitude, has been shown to vary as a function of rated valence and arousal (Meagher et al., 2001). Moreover, the hedonic response to IAPS pictures has been related to opioid neurotransmission, showing that remifentanil, a µ-opioid receptor agonist, increases the experienced pleasantness of neutral pictures (Gospic et al., 2008).

Still, it was not without reluctance, that I decided to use IAPS pictures for pleasure induction. For me, these pictures have an American and outdated '80ies patina' and I doubted their hedonic impact. However, during the experiments, and in pre-tests, not reported here, subjective ratings on the degree of induced pleasantness were comparable to prior norms. Several studies have confirmed that the valence of an emotional state determines the *direction* of pain modulation: pleasant states decrease, while unpleasant states increase pain perception (Meagher et al., 2001; Rhudy et al., 2008; Wiech and Tracey, 2009). The *magnitude* of modulation is however determined by the level of arousal, suggesting that arousal modulates the level of activation of both the appetitive and aversive systems. As discussed in chapter 6.4 the presentation of pleasant pictures, mostly erotic in nature, within the experimental setting – the experimenters sitting nearby, though behind a partition – most probably lowered arousal and endogenous opioid release. In designing and executing the *opioid-study* I realized how difficult it is to induce highly pleasant and at the same time highly arousing pleasant states, particularly in experimental settings. While pictures of a shredded hand or mutilated bodies evoke instantaneously highly arousing negative feelings in almost everyone, except maybe for surgeons, specialists in forensic medicine, or psychotics, the picture of an erotic couple may elicit a spectrum of emotions in different degrees of valence and arousal. It appears that we are primed to respond equivocally to aversive stimuli, while our response to appetitive stimuli is much more shaped by context, individual memories, desires, and tempers. Moreover, what intrigues me, are ambivalent feelings, as for example melancholy. Although the word does not exist, we all know what 'ambiarousal' describes. There are sometimes moments in life, when we experience feelings in the appropriate valence, as we are for example sad or angry when loosing a loved one, or joyful and proud when passing a difficult challenge, but not as intense or arousing as we would expect ourselves to feel. Absolute and overwhelmingly pleasurable or joyful emotional states – that are not induced by sex or drugs – are once in a blue moon in adult life.

*Pleasure in the brain*

> "Modern science begins to understand pleasure
> as a potential component of salutogenesis"
> – Tobias Esch & George B. Stefano, 2004

What is it about pleasure research that might make one feel slightly awkward? Leknes and Tracey argument in their Nature neuroscience review on pain and pleasure "The Calvinistic focus on moderation, or even abstinence, of pleasure has deep roots in Western culture and is powerfully connected with shame" (Leknes and Tracey, 2008). The belief in shame and stoicism and the focus on pathogenic processes in medicine might account for the vast number of publications on depression, anxiety and other mental disorders, and the neglect of salutogenic functions of positive sensations and mind states like satisfaction and contentment and feelings of joy and bliss (Esch and Stefano, 2004). In these last years, affective neuroscientists have increasingly turned their interest from studying disease mechanisms in the ill brain towards the study of the healthy and well-tempered brain. Believe it or not, there are even publications on the 'neurobiology of wisdom' and 'pragmatic knowledge of life' (Meeks and Jeste, 2009). Pleasure can foster cognition, productivity, and health[36] but clearly enough, it can also promote addiction and other negative behaviours. Esch et

---

[36] Psychoneuroimmunology provides a lot of insight on the interactions between emotion and the activity of the immune system. Opioid pentapeptides stimulate for example cytokine release and immunocyte chemotaxis (Stefano et al., 1998).

al. term it as 'motivational toxicity' and emphasize that the concrete outcome of pleasant experiences may be, evidently, a question of dose (Esch and Stefano, 2004). Neurobiological research on pleasure processes in the brain has tried to face the challenge of understanding how core processes of pleasure, originating from activity across widespread brain systems, are converted to conscious pleasure (Berridge, 2003). How can a core process for positive emotional reaction in the nucleus accumbens shell interact with voluntary cognitive regulation in cortical brain systems, or pain processing? This brings us back to the opioid circuitry, since positive emotional reactions to sweetness for example, appear to be mediated in the nucleus accumbens by this neurotransmitter system (Pecina, 2008). We have also seen that results from studies using microinjections of morphine in specific rat brain regions are one thing, and results from pleasure induction followed by neurotransmitter antagonisation in human volunteers another. Still, there is another important question that should not be forgotten: is sensory pleasure from food intake or drugs comparable with pleasure, originating from being in love, social joy, sex, parenthood, intellectual pleasure from art, literature, or music, humour, money gain, social approval, and adventure? Or in other words, how many types of pleasure are there in the brain? I would like to sum up with a citation of Berridge that I really enjoy: "The search for understanding of how positive affective reactions are generated by the brain will long remain a source of cerebral pleasure for those who have a taste for that sort of thing" (Berridge, 2003).

## *Mind as real as matter?*

> "The physical pain alone was terrible. I always used to think
> the expression 'a broken heart' was just a metaphor.
> But it felt as if I was having a heart attack."
> – Bob Geldof (on the end of his 19-year relationship)

It has long been common in diverse human cultures for people to talk about loss of a loved one in terms of painful feelings. This seems to be more than a semantic metaphor. Recent neurobiological research indicates that reactions to rejection and loss are mediated by aspects of the physical pain system (Eisenberger et al., 2003; Panksepp, 2003). Panksepp and colleagues were the first to suggest that brain circuits for separation distress represent an evolutionary elaboration of a pain network (Panksepp et al., 1978). Low doses of morphine indeed reduce the separation distress cries of isolated rat pups, primates, dogs, guinea pigs, and birds (Macdonald and Leary, 2005). Also human brain bases of social pain are similar to those of physical pain, as demonstrated in the study, where grieving over the death of a loved one deactivated µ-opioid neurotransmission (Zubieta et al., 2003). It is interesting to note, that these brain bases are homologous with those of other mammals (Eisenberger et al., 2003). Thus, the brain may treat abstract social experiences and concrete physical experiences as more similar than traditional mind-body separation views imply. The findings that the hurtfulness of social pain and physical pain both emerge in the same brain areas point toward common motivational importance ensuring mammalian survival by preventing a disruption of social connections and engendering pro-social behaviours. Likewise, pleasurable experiences are augmented in social contexts (Esch and Stefano, 2004). Not only, is eating and drinking more fun in a circle of friends, social rewards even activate the same reward network as desirable foods and drinks do (Lieberman and Eisenberger, 2009). A joy shared is a joy doubled. All of these results add to a growing body of literature suggesting that the common circuits, neuroanatomical areas and neurotransmitter systems – such as the opioid system (Bodnar, 2008) – that are involved in emotion, pain and stress may be related "not simply to a shared circuit but to underlying dimensional factors that transcend the traditional categorical separation of physical and emotional functions, responses and disease processes" (Ribeiro et al., 2005).

*Molecular feelings*

> "Mein Herz tanzt!
> Uhuhu
> und jedes Molekül
> bewegt sich!"
> – MIA, Tanz der Moleküle. 2006

The ease with which nowadays neuroscientists rhetorically transgress the traditional categories of mind and body might be strongly influenced by the neurobiological and pharmacological discoveries made in the 20$^{th}$ century. When Albert Hofmann first synthesized LSD (Lysergic acid diethylamide) in 1938, brain research was in its infancy (Nichols, 2006). Already a few years later its profound effects on the brain promoted the view that the newly identified neurotransmitter serotonin, similar in molecular structure, plays an important role in mental illnesses, such as loss of pleasure and feelings of hopelessness in depressive patients, and gave birth to the field of neuroscience. At the time, the idea was extremely controversial and not widely embraced, still the implications were enormous (Nichols, 2006). Today, there are a number of established drugs that interact with serotonin receptors, alleviating depression, schizophrenia, and pain.

Doubtlessly, emotions and feelings are – if not completely based – than at least influenced by the brain's neurochemistry. I have cited various studies on opioids and dopamine, and there are countless other studies on the relationship between the regulation and dysregulation of other endogenous molecules and mental phenomena. Still, the outcome of the *opioid study* comforts me in a certain way. There is no 1:1 relation between a chemical pathway and a certain feeling. The hedonic response to pleasant stimuli and pleasure-related analgesia, as measured in heat pain tolerance, has shown to be robust to blockade of opioid neurotransmission, while at the same time subjective pain ratings increased. These results suggest an intricate interplay of different top-down processes, which might be based on discrete time scales and feed-back mechanisms. Indeed, research on the genetic and functional diversity of the opioid receptor classes exemplifies, instead of a simple on/off, a complex pattern of signalling wherein multiple, co-ordinately secreted peptides interact with multiple receptors to effect intricate regulation of pain and other phenomena (McNally and Akil, 2002).

## 7.2 Summary and conclusion

> "The Socratic dictum *know thyself* necessarily involves being in tune not only with one's thoughts and outside reality but also with the subtle or more severe emotional reactions, which are primary evaluative tools of meaning and value."
> – Saulo C. Ribeiro et al., 2005

Pain is a highly subjective experience and not necessarily related linearly to a nociceptive input. Since not only genetic, or pathological factors shape individual pain experience, but also memory, motivation, thoughts, beliefs and emotions, it is an intriguing study object for understanding 'body and mind' interactions.

The first methodological study (*psychophysics study*) of this thesis demonstrated that experimental heat pain delivered to the volar forearm is a suitable way to investigate individual pain threshold and tolerance and can be used in experimental or clinical settings, when comparing for example patients and healthy volunteers. Pain threshold and pain tolerance did not differ within and across forearm sites. Moreover, there were high correlations of threshold and tolerance values across sites and side of stimulation, suggesting a rather evenly distributed density of heat pain receptors amongst the sites in the forearms.

In the second study (*role-identity study*) the focus was turned to contextual and emotional aspects of pain perception. As hypothesized results showed that changing self-perceived identity into a *hero/heroine* or a *faint-heart* indeed significantly modulated pain. Pain was better tolerated whenever the role identity was embedded in an unavoidable, unpleasant context, but which confered pain a meaningful and thus suitable character. Subjective ratings suggested that the self-image changed emotions accordingly, which in turn affected intensity and quality of pain perception. The spectrum of positive versus negative feelings was most probably combined with the presence or absence of the willingness to endure pain.

The third study (*opioid study*) approached the neural underpinnings of emotional pain modulation. Since evidence from placebo studies robustly showed how expectation and desire for pain relief activates top-down pain inhibitory processes emphasising the role played by endogenous opioids in the interactions between cognition, emotion and sensory experiences (Ribeiro et al., 2005), this neurotransmitter system was addressed. It was hypothesized that during positive emotional states opioidergic neurotransmission is enhanced, which in turn leads to alleviated pain perception. However, despite complete $\mu$-opioid receptor antagonisation with naloxone, pleasant picture viewing succeeded in eliciting positive emotional states and concomitant pleasure-related analgesia. In contrast, subjective pain ratings increased after naloxone administration, suggesting that the appraisal of noxious heat stimuli was opioid-sensitive. These results revealed that besides opioid neurotransmission, non-opioid mediated circuits play a major role in the regulation of pain and emotions.

The findings of this thesis clearly demonstrate that pain is a dynamic experience, by which noxious stimuli are permanently modulated and reevaluated within a broader context of the individual and its interaction with the environment. Hereby, emotions, such as pleasure, braveness, or helplessness, expectations, past experiences, and the value of pain in comparison to other motivations, lead to a constant resetting of pain tolerance based on the interaction of intricate pain-modulatory circuits. The acknowledgment of the organism as a unity, where mental phenomena have physical consequences, and vice versa physical events affect the mental state, shapes our understanding of salutogenesis and bodily and emotional homeostasis. It should therefore be of great value for both the care of pain patients and also the individual and clinical management of other challenges of life.

## 7.3 Outlook

The results of the role-identity study have wide implications for the treatment of clinical pain patients. Doubtlessly, it is easier for a healthy, painfree volunteer to be a *hero/heroine* in order to tolerate an acute painful stimulus, than it is for a patient to endure constant debilitating pain. Still, meaningfulness of pain, as for instance propagated in religious communities and used as an aspect of the *hero/heroine* role-play, can be a strong mean to cope with hurtful events. A consequence of this is to test our role-plays as therapeutic means, which by manipulating self-perceived role identity may decrease pain in chronic patients. In cooperation with Kathi Thieme, PhD, such a study is planned at the Central Institute for Mental Health Mannheim. The study will investigate the influence of role identity and associated emotions on pain perception and processing as well as on pain behaviours in ninety patients with fibromyalgia-syndrome compared to twenty healthy controls. A major scientific challenge is the understanding of endogenous pain systems as a form of "endogenous healthcare system" (Enck et al., 2008). I think that the information one can gain from measuring behavioural parameters in humans, such as pain tolerance and subjective ratings, after neurotransmitter antagonisation is of general character and allows only modest conclusions on the underlying neurobiology. New insights of opioidergic, dopaminergic, cannabionidergic, and serotonergic function in acute and chronic pain processing might, however, come from the *combination* of these kind of studies together with animal data and the capacity to image neurotransmitters via molecular imaging in humans. The synthesis of this data will doubtlessly lead to advances in drug development by detecting new target structures and mechanisms. Moreover, knowledge on cognitive and emotional modulation of bodily functions is already shaping our concept of drug actions, as for example a new drug might have no analgesic properties, but enhance placebo activated endogenous opioid release (Colloca and Benedetti, 2005), and will consequently impact the design of clinical trials.

# 8
# Appendix

## 8.1 References

Amanzio, M., and Benedetti, F. (1999). Neuropharmacological dissection of placebo analgesia: expectation-activated opioid systems versus conditioning-activated specific subsystems. J Neurosci *19*, 484-494.

Amanzio, M., Pollo, A., Maggi, G., and Benedetti, F. (2001). Response variability to analgesics: a role for non-specific activation of endogenous opioids. Pain *90*, 205-215.

Apkarian, A.V., Bushnell, M.C., Treede, R.D., and Zubieta, J.K. (2005). Human brain mechanisms of pain perception and regulation in health and disease. Eur J Pain *9*, 463-484.

Arzneimittel-Kompendium (2006). Monographie von Naloxon OrPha (OrPha Swiss GmbH, Zürich) (Basel, Documed AG).

Avenanti, A., Bueti, D., Galati, G., and Aglioti, S.M. (2005). Transcranial magnetic stimulation highlights the sensorimotor side of empathy for pain. Nat Neurosci *8*, 955-960.

Aydede, M., ed. (2005). Pain: New essays on its nature and the methodology of its study (Cambridge, MA: MIT Press).

Bantick, S.J., Wise, R.G., Ploghaus, A., Clare, S., Smith, S.M., and Tracey, I. (2002). Imaging how attention modulates pain in humans using functional MRI. Brain *125*, 310-319.

Bar, K.J., Brehm, S., Boettger, M.K., Boettger, S., Wagner, G., and Sauer, H. (2005). Pain perception in major depression depends on pain modality. Pain *117*, 97-103.

Bar, K.J., Greiner, W., Letsch, A., Kobele, R., and Sauer, H. (2003). Influence of gender and hemispheric lateralization on heat pain perception in major depression. Journal of psychiatric research *37*, 345-353.

Basbaum, A.I., and Fields, H.L. (1984). Endogenous pain control systems: brainstem spinal pathways and endorphin circuitry. Annu Rev Neurosci *7*, 309-338.

Becerra, L., Breiter, H.C., Wise, R., Gonzalez, R.G., and Borsook, D. (2001). Reward circuitry activation by noxious thermal stimuli. Neuron *32*, 927-946.

Bencherif, B., Fuchs, P.N., Sheth, R., Dannals, R.F., Campbell, J.N., and Frost, J.J. (2002). Pain activation of human supraspinal opioid pathways as demonstrated by [11C]-carfentanil and positron emission tomography (PET). Pain *99*, 589-598.

Benedetti, F. (1996). The opposite effects of the opiate antagonist naloxone and the cholecystokinin antagonist proglumide on placebo analgesia. Pain *64*, 535-543.

Benedetti, F., Mayberg, H.S., Wager, T.D., Stohler, C.S., and Zubieta, J.K. (2005). Neurobiological mechanisms of the placebo effect. J Neurosci *25*, 10390-10402.

Berridge, K.C. (2003). Pleasures of the brain. Brain and cognition *52*, 106-128.

Bingel, U., Quante, M., Knab, R., Bromm, B., Weiller, C., and Buchel, C. (2003). Single trial fMRI reveals significant contralateral bias in responses to laser pain within thalamus and somatosensory cortices. Neuroimage *18*, 740-748.

Blanchard, C., Blanchard, R., Fellous, J.M., Guimaraes, F.S., Irwin, W., Ledoux, J.E., McGaugh, J.L., Rosen, J.B., Schenberg, L.C., Volchan, E., and Da Cunha, C. (2001). The brain decade in debate: III. Neurobiology of emotion. Braz J Med Biol Res *34*, 283-293.

Blumenthal, T.D., Cuthbert, B.N., Filion, D.L., Hackley, S., Lipp, O.V., and van Boxtel, A. (2005). Committee report: Guidelines for human startle eyeblink electromyographic studies. Psychophysiology *42*, 1-15.

Bodnar, R.J. (2008). Endogenous opiates and behavior: 2007. Peptides *29*, 2292-2375.

Boecker, H., Sprenger, T., Spilker, M.E., Henriksen, G., Koppenhoefer, M., Wagner, K.J., Valet, M., Berthele, A., and Tolle, T.R. (2008). The runner's high: opioidergic mechanisms in the human brain. Cereb Cortex *18*, 2523-2531.

Boly, M., Faymonville, M.E., Schnakers, C., Peigneux, P., Lambermont, B., Phillips, C., Lancellotti, P., Luxen, A., Lamy, M., Moonen, G., *et al.* (2008). Perception of pain in the minimally conscious state with PET activation: an observational study. Lancet Neurol *7*, 1013-1020.

Borras, M.C., Becerra, L., Ploghaus, A., Gostic, J.M., DaSilva, A., Gonzalez, R.G., and Borsook, D. (2004). fMRI measurement of CNS responses to naloxone infusion and subsequent mild noxious thermal stimuli in healthy volunteers. J Neurophysiol *91*, 2723-2733.

Bradley, M.M., Codispoti, M., and Lang, P.J. (2006). A multi-process account of startle modulation during affective perception. Psychophysiology *43*, 486-497.

Breivik, H., Collett, B., Ventafridda, V., Cohen, R., and Gallacher, D. (2006). Survey of chronic pain in Europe: prevalence, impact on daily life, and treatment. Eur J Pain *10*, 287-333.

Brownstein, M.J. (1993). A brief history of opiates, opioid peptides, and opioid receptors. Proc Natl Acad Sci U S A *90*, 5391-5393.

Bruehl, S., Burns, J.W., Chung, O.Y., Ward, P., and Johnson, B. (2002). Anger and pain sensitivity in chronic low back pain patients and pain-free controls: the role of endogenous opioids. Pain *99*, 223-233.

Bullmore, E., and Sporns, O. (2009). Complex brain networks: graph theoretical analysis of structural and functional systems. Nat Rev Neurosci *10*, 186-198.

Burgdorf, J., and Panksepp, J. (2006). The neurobiology of positive emotions. Neurosci Biobehav Rev *30*, 173-187.

Calder, A.J., Lawrence, A.D., and Young, A.W. (2001). Neuropsychology of fear and loathing. Nat Rev Neurosci *2*, 352-363.

Cannon, W.B. (1927). The James-Lange theory of emotions: a critical examination and an alternative theory. Am J Psychol *39*, 106-124.

Casey, K.L. (1999). Forebrain mechanisms of nociception and pain: analysis through imaging. Proc Natl Acad Sci U S A *96*, 7668-7674.

Chapman, L.J., and Chapman, J.P. (1987). The measurement of handedness. Brain and cognition *6*, 175-183.

Colloca, L., and Benedetti, F. (2005). Placebos and painkillers: is mind as real as matter? Nat Rev Neurosci *6*, 545-552.

Craig, A.D. (2003). A new view of pain as a homeostatic emotion. Trends Neurosci *26*, 303-307.

Dalgleish, T. (2004). The emotional brain. Nat Rev Neurosci *5*, 583-589.

Damasio, A.R. (1994). Descartes' error: Emotion, reason, and the human brain (New York: Putnam).

Damasio, A.R. (1998). Emotion in the perspective of an integrated nervous system. Brain Res Brain Res Rev *26*, 83-86.

Darwin, C. (1872/1998). The expression of the emotions in man and animals (New York: Oxford University Press).

Davidson, R.J., Scherer, K.R., and Goldsmith, H.H. (2003). Handbook of Affective Sciences (New York: Oxford University Press).

de Quervain, D.J., Fischbacher, U., Treyer, V., Schellhammer, M., Schnyder, U., Buck, A., and Fehr, E. (2004). The neural basis of altruistic punishment. Science *305*, 1254-1258.

de Wied, M., and Verbaten, M.N. (2001). Affective pictures processing, attention, and pain tolerance. Pain *90*, 163-172.

Demmerling, C., and Landweer, H. (2007). Philosophie der Gefühle: Von Achtung bis Zorn (Stuttgart: Metzler).

Dickenson, A.H. (1997). Plasticity: implications for opioid and other pharmacological interventions in specific pain states. Behav Brain Sci *20*, 392-403; discussion 435-513.

Dolan, R.J. (2002). Emotion, cognition, and behavior. Science *298*, 1191-1194.

Duden (2004). Duden: Das Synonymwörterbuch, Vol 8 (Mannheim: Dudenverlag).

Edwards, R., Augustson, E.M., and Fillingim, R. (2000). Sex-specific effects of pain-related anxiety on adjustment to chronic pain. Clin. J. Pain *16*, 46-53.

Eisenberger, N.I., Lieberman, M.D., and Williams, K.D. (2003). Does Rejection Hurt? An fMRI Study of Social Exclusion. Science *302*, 290-292.

Ekman, P., and Davidson, R.J., eds. (1994). The nature of emotion: Fundamental questions (New York: Oxford University Press).

Enck, P., Benedetti, F., and Schedlowski, M. (2008). New insights into the placebo and nocebo responses. Neuron *59*, 195-206.

Esch, T., and Stefano, G.B. (2004). The neurobiology of pleasure, reward processes, addiction and their health implications. Neuro Endocrinol Lett *25*, 235-251.

Fichna, J., Janecka, A., Costentin, J., and Do Rego, J.C. (2007). The endomorphin system and its evolving neurophysiological role. Pharmacol Rev *59*, 88-123.

Fields, H. (2004). State-dependent opioid control of pain. Nat Rev Neurosci *5*, 565-575.

Fields, H.L. (2007). Understanding how opioids contribute to reward and analgesia. Reg Anesth Pain Med *32*, 242-246.

Fields, H.L., and Levine, F.M. (1984). Placebo analgesia – a role for endorphins? Trends Neurosci *7*, 271-273.

Fillingim, R.B., Maixner, W., Kincaid, S., and Silva, S. (1998). Sex differences in temporal summation but not sensory-discriminative processing of thermal pain. Pain *75*, 121-127.

Fillingim, R.B., Ness, T.J., Glover, T.L., Campbell, C.M., Hastie, B.A., Price, D.D., and Staud, R. (2005). Morphine responses and experimental pain: sex differences in side effects and cardiovascular responses but not analgesia. J Pain *6*, 116-124.

Flor, H., Birbaumer, N., Schulz, R., Grusser, S.M., and Mucha, R.F. (2002). Pavlovian conditioning of opioid and nonopioid pain inhibitory mechanisms in humans. Eur J Pain *6*, 395-402.

Folkers, G., and Wittwer, A. (2007). Drug design and emotion. AIP Conf Proc *958*, 3-8.

Ford, G.K., and Finn, D.P. (2008). Clinical correlates of stress-induced analgesia: evidence from pharmacological studies. Pain *140*, 3-7.

Geers, A.L., Wellman, J.A., Helfer, S.G., Fowler, S.L., and France, C.R. (2008). Dispositional optimism and thoughts of well-being determine sensitivity to an experimental pain task. Ann Behav Med *36*, 304-313.

Gladwell, M. (2005). Blink: The power of thinking without thinking (New York: Little Brown and Company).

Goldberg, I.E., Rossi, G.C., Letchworth, S.R., Mathis, J.P., Ryan-Moro, J., Leventhal, L., Su, W., Emmel, D., Bolan, E.A., and Pasternak, G.W. (1998). Pharmacological characterization of endomorphin-1 and endomorphin-2 in mouse brain. J Pharmacol Exp Ther *286*, 1007-1013.

Goldie, P. (2000). The emotions: A philosophical exploration (Oxford: Clarendon Press).

Gospic, K., Gunnarsson, T., Fransson, P., Ingvar, M., Lindefors, N., and Petrovic, P. (2008). Emotional perception modulated by an opioid and a cholecystokinin agonist. Psychopharmacology (Berl) *197*, 295-307.

Gracely, R.H., Dubner, R., Wolskee, P.J., and Deeter, W.R. (1983). Placebo and naloxone can alter post-surgical pain by separate mechanisms. Nature *306*, 264-265.

Grandjean, D., Sander, D., Pourtois, G., Schwartz, S., Seghier, M.L., Scherer, K.R., and Vuilleumier, P. (2005). The voices of wrath: brain responses to angry prosody in meaningless speech. Nat. Neurosci. *8*, 145-146.

Granot, M., Granovsky, Y., Sprecher, E., Nir, R.R., and Yarnitsky, D. (2006). Contact heat-evoked temporal summation: tonic versus repetitive-phasic stimulation. Pain *122*, 295-305.

Granot, M., Sprecher, E., and Yarnitsky, D. (2003). Psychophysics of phasic and tonic heat pain stimuli by quantitative sensory testing in healthy subjects. Eur J Pain *7*, 139-143.

Grevert, P., Albert, L.H., and Goldstein, A. (1983). Partial antagonism of placebo analgesia by naloxone. Pain *16*, 129-143.

Hagander, L.G., Midani, H.A., Kuskowski, M.A., and Parry, G.J. (2000). Quantitative sensory testing: effect of site and skin temperature on thermal thresholds. Clin Neurophysiol *111*, 17-22.

Haythornthwaite, J.A., and Benrud-Larson, L.M. (2000). Psychological aspects of neuropathic pain. Clin J Pain *16*, S101-105.

Hermann, I. (2006). Schmerzarten: Prolegomena einer Ästhetik des Schmerzes in Literatur, Musik und Psychoanalyse (Heidelberg: Winter).

Hill, R.G. (1981). The status of naloxone in the identification of pain control mechanisms operated by endogenous opioids. Neurosci Lett *21*, 217-222.

Horvath, G. (2000). Endomorphin-1 and endomorphin-2: pharmacology of the selective endogenous mu-opioid receptor agonists. Pharmacol Ther *88*, 437-463.

Hsieh, J.C., Stone-Elander, S., and Ingvar, M. (1999). Anticipatory coping of pain expressed in the human anterior cingulate cortex: a positron emission tomography study. Neurosci Lett *262*, 61-64.

Ingvar, M. (1999). Pain and functional imaging. Philos Trans R Soc Lond B Biol Sci *354*, 1347-1358.

James, W. (1884). What is an emotion? Mind *9*, 188-205.

Janssen, S.A., and Arntz, A. (1996). Anxiety and pain: attentional and endorphinergic influences. Pain *66*, 145-150.

Johnstone, T., and Scherer, K.R. (2000). Vocal Communication of Emotion. In Handbook of Emotions, M. Lewis, and J.M. Haviland-Jones, eds. (New York: Guilford Press), pp. 220-235.

Jones, A.K., Cunningham, V.J., Ha-Kawa, S., Fujiwara, T., Luthra, S.K., Silva, S., Derbyshire, S., and Jones, T. (1994). Changes in central opioid receptor binding in relation to inflammation and pain in patients with rheumatoid arthritis. Br J Rheumatol *33*, 909-916.

Junghofer, M., Sabatinelli, D., Bradley, M.M., Schupp, H.T., Elbert, T.R., and Lang, P.J. (2006). Fleeting images: rapid affect discrimination in the visual cortex. Neuroreport *17*, 225-229.

Kallai, I., Barke, A., and Voss, U. (2004). The effects of experimenter characteristics on pain reports in women and men. Pain *112*, 142-147.

Kalter-Leibovici, O., Yosipovitch, G., Gabbay, U., Yarnitsky, D., and Karp, M. (2001). Factor analysis of thermal and vibration thresholds in young patients with Type 1 diabetes mellitus. Diabet Med *18*, 213-217.

Keogh, E., and Herdenfeldt, M. (2002). Gender, coping and the perception of pain. Pain *97*, 195-201.

Knabl, J., Witschi, R., Hosl, K., Reinold, H., Zeilhofer, U.B., Ahmadi, S., Brockhaus, J., Sergejeva, M., Hess, A., Brune, K., *et al.* (2008). Reversal of pathological pain through specific spinal GABAA receptor subtypes. Nature *451*, 330-334.

Koepp, M.J., Hammers, A., Lawrence, A.D., Asselin, M.C., Grasby, P.M., and Bench, C.J. (2009). Evidence for endogenous opioid release in the amygdala during positive emotion. Neuroimage *44*, 252-256.

Koob, G.F., and Le Moal, M. (1997). Drug abuse: hedonic homeostatic dysregulation. Science *278*, 52-58.

Koyama, T., McHaffie, J.G., Laurienti, P.J., and Coghill, R.C. (2005). The subjective experience of pain: where expectations become reality. Proc Natl Acad Sci U S A *102*, 12950-12955.

Kuba, T., and Quinones-Jenab, V. (2005). The role of female gonadal hormones in behavioral sex differences in persistent and chronic pain: clinical versus preclinical studies. Brain Res Bull *66*, 179-188.

Kut, E., Schaffner, N., Wittwer, A., Candia, V., Brockmann, M., Storck, C., and Folkers, G. (2007). Changes in self-perceived role identity modulate pain perception. Pain *131*, 191-201.

Kut, E., Candia, V., von Overbeck, J., Pok, J., Fink, D., Folkers, G. (2011). Pleasure-related analgesia activates opioid-insensitive circuits. J Neurosci *31*, 4148-4153.

LaMotte, R.H., and Campbell, J.N. (1978). Comparison of responses of warm and nociceptive C-fiber afferents in monkey with human judgments of thermal pain. J Neurophysiol *41*, 509-528.

Lang, P.J. (1980). Behavioral treatment and bio-behavioral assessment: computer applications. In Technology in mental health care delivery system, J.B. Sidowski, J.H. Johnson, and E.A. Williams, eds. (Norwood, NJ: Ablex), pp. 119-137.

Lang, P.J. (1995). The emotion probe. Studies of motivation and attention. Am Psychol *50*, 372-385.

Lang, P.J., Bradley, M.M., and Cuthbert, B.N. (1990). Emotion, attention, and the startle reflex. Psychol Rev *97*, 377-395.

Lang, P.J., Bradley, M.M., and Cuthbert, B.N. (2004). International affective picture system (IAPS): Affective ratings of pictures and instruction manual. Technical Report A-6. (Gainesville, FL: University of Florida).

Laruelle, M. (2000). Imaging synaptic neurotransmission with in vivo binding competition techniques: a critical review. J Cereb Blood Flow Metab *20*, 423-451.

LeDoux, J.E. (2000). Emotion circuits in the brain. Annu Rev Neurosci *23*, 155-184.

Leknes, S., and Tracey, I. (2008). A common neurobiology for pain and pleasure. Nat Rev Neurosci *9*, 314-320.

Levine, F.M., and De Simone, L.L. (1991). The effects of experimenter gender on pain report in male and female subjects. Pain *44*, 69-72.

Levine, J.D., Gordon, N.C., and Fields, H.L. (1978). The mechanism of placebo analgesia. Lancet *2*, 654-657.

Lewis, M., and Haviland-Jones, J.M. (2000). Handbook of Emotions, Second edn (New York: Guilford Press).

Li, Z.H., Shan, L.D., Jiang, X.H., Guo, S.Y., Yu, G.D., Hisamitsu, T., and Yin, Q.Z. (2001). Analgesic effect of endomorphin-1. Acta Pharmacol Sin *22*, 976-980.

Lieberman, M.D., and Eisenberger, N.I. (2009). Pains and pleasures of social life. Science *323*, 890-891.

Lieberman, M.D., Eisenberger, N.I., Crockett, M.J., Tom, S.M., Pfeifer, J.H., and Way, B.M. (2007). Putting feelings into words: affect labeling disrupts amygdala activity in response to affective stimuli. Psychol Sci *18*, 421-428.

Long, D.A. (1994). Hand differences and reported intensity of nociceptive stimuli. Percept Mot Skills *79*, 411-417.

Ludlow, C. (1987). Laryngeal Function in Phonation and Respiration: Vocal Fold Physiology Series (Boston: College Hill).

Lugo, M., Isturiz, G., Lara, C., Garcia, N., and Eblen-Zaijur, A. (2002). Sensory lateralization in pain subjective perception for noxious heat stimulus. Somatosens Mot Res *19*, 207-212.

Luo, X., Pietrobon, R., Sun, S.X., Liu, G.G., and Hey, L. (2004). Estimates and patterns of direct health care expenditures among individuals with back pain in the United States. Spine (Phila Pa 1976) *29*, 79-86.

Macdonald, G., and Leary, M.R. (2005). Why does social exclusion hurt? The relationship between social and physical pain. Psychol Bull *131*, 202-223.

Maclean, P.D. (1952). Some psychiatric implications of physiological studies on frontotemporal portion of limbic system (visceral brain). Electroencephalogr Clin Neurophysiol *4*, 407-418.

Magnusson, J.E., and Fisher, K. (2000). The involvement of dopamine in nociception: the role of D(1) and D(2) receptors in the dorsolateral striatum. Brain Res *855*, 260-266.

Marchand, S., and Arsenault, P. (2002). Odors modulate pain perception: a gender-specific effect. Physiology & behavior *76*, 251-256.

Matthes, H.W., Smadja, C., Valverde, O., Vonesch, J.L., Foutz, A.S., Boudinot, E., Denavit-Saubie, M., Severini, C., Negri, L., Roques, B.P.*, et al.* (1998). Activity of the delta-opioid receptor is partially reduced, whereas activity of the kappa-receptor is maintained in mice lacking the mu-receptor. J Neurosci *18*, 7285-7295.

McNally, G.P., and Akil, H. (2002). Opioid Peptides and their Receptors: Overview and Function in Pain Modulation. In Neuropsychopharmacology: The Fifth Generation of Progress, K.L. Davis, and D. Charney, eds. (New York: Lippincott & Williams).

Meador, K.J., Ray, P.G., Day, L., Ghelani, H., and Loring, D.W. (1998). Physiology of somatosensory perception: cerebral lateralization and extinction. Neurology *51*, 721-727.

Meagher, M.W., Arnau, R.C., and Rhudy, J.L. (2001). Pain and emotion: effects of affective picture modulation. Psychosom Med *63*, 79-90.

Meeks, T.W., and Jeste, D.V. (2009). Neurobiology of wisdom: a literature overview. Arch Gen Psychiatry *66*, 355-365.

Meh, D., and Denislic, M. (1994). Quantitative assessment of thermal and pain sensitivity. J Neurol Sci *127*, 164-169.

Melzack, R. (1975). The McGill Pain Questionnaire: major properties and scoring methods. Pain *1*, 277-299.

Melzack, R. (2008). The future of pain. Nat Rev Drug Discov *7*, 629.

Melzack, R., and Casey, K.L. (1968). Sensory, motivational, and central control determinants of pain. In The Skin senses, D.R. Kenshalo, ed. (Springfield: Charles C. Thomas), pp. 423-443.

Melzack, R., Wall, P.D., and Ty, T.C. (1982). Acute pain in an emergency clinic: latency of onset and descriptor patterns related to different injuries. Pain *14*, 33-43.

Mendoza, E. (1998). Acoustic analysis of induced vocal stress by means of cognitive workload tasks. J. Voice *12*, 263-273.

Merskey, H., and Bogduk, N., eds. (1994). Classification of Chronic Pain. Descriptions of Chronic Pain Syndromes and Definitions of Pain Terms, 2 edn (Seattle: IASP Press).

Millan, M.J. (2002). Descending control of pain. Prog Neurobiol *66*, 355-474.

Miller, G.A. (2003). The cognitive revolution: a historical perspective. Trends Cogn Sci *7*, 141-144.

Morris, D.B. (1994). Geschichte des Schmerzes (Frankfurt am Main: Insel Verlag).

Nagel, T. (1974). What is it like to be a bat. Philosophical Review *83*, 435-450.

Narcan (2001). http://www.fda.gov/cder/foi/label/2002/16636slr054lbl.pdf.

Nichols, D. (2006). LSD: cultural revolution and medical advances. Chemistry World *3*.

Niedenthal, P.M. (2007). Embodying emotion. Science *316*, 1002-1005.

Oldfield, R.C. (1971). The assessment and analysis of handedness: the Edinburgh inventory. Neuropsychologia *9*, 97-113.

Panksepp, J. (2003). Feeling the pain of social loss. Science *302*, 237-239.

Panksepp, J. (2005). On the neuro-evolutionary nature of social pain, support, and empathy. In Pain: New essays on its nature and the methodology of its study, M. Aydede, ed. (Cambridge, MA: MIT Press).

Panksepp, J., Herman, B., Conner, R., Bishop, P., and Scott, J.P. (1978). The biology of social attachments: opiates alleviate separation distress. Biol Psychiatry *13*, 607-618.

Papez, J.W. (1937). A proposed mechanism of emotion. Arch Neurol Psychiatry *38*, 725-743.

Pauli, P., Wiedemann, G., and Nickola, M. (1999). Pain sensitivity, cerebral laterality, and negative affect. Pain *80*, 359-364.

Pecina, S. (2008). Opioid reward 'liking' and 'wanting' in the nucleus accumbens. Physiology & behavior *94*, 675-680.

Pessoa, L. (2008). On the relationship between emotion and cognition. Nat Rev Neurosci *9*, 148-158.

Petrovic, P., Kalso, E., Petersson, K.M., and Ingvar, M. (2002). Placebo and opioid analgesia-- imaging a shared neuronal network. Science *295*, 1737-1740.

Petrovic, P., Petersson, K.M., Ghatan, P.H., Stone-Elander, S., and Ingvar, M. (2000). Pain-related cerebral activation is altered by a distracting cognitive task. Pain *85*, 19-30.

Petrovic, P., Pleger, B., Seymour, B., Kloppel, S., De Martino, B., Critchley, H., and Dolan, R.J. (2008). Blocking central opiate function modulates hedonic impact and anterior cingulate response to rewards and losses. J Neurosci *28*, 10509-10516.

Peyron, R., Garcia-Larrea, L., Gregoire, M.C., Costes, N., Convers, P., Lavenne, F., Mauguiere, F., Michel, D., and Laurent, B. (1999). Haemodynamic brain responses to acute pain in humans: sensory and attentional networks. Brain *122 ( Pt 9)*, 1765-1780.

Phelps, E.A. (2006). Emotion and cognition: insights from studies of the human amygdala. Annu Rev Psychol *57*, 27-53.

Ploghaus, A., Tracey, I., Gati, J.S., Clare, S., Menon, R.S., Matthews, P.M., and Rawlins, J.N. (1999). Dissociating pain from its anticipation in the human brain. Science *284*, 1979-1981.

Price, D.D. (2000). Psychological and neural mechanisms of the affective dimension of pain. Science *288*, 1769-1772.

Price, D.D. (2002). Central neural mechanisms that interrelate sensory and affective dimensions of pain. Mol Interv *2*, 392-403, 339.

Price, D.D., McGrath, P.A., Rafii, A., and Buckingham, B. (1983). The validation of visual analogue scales as ratio scale measures for chronic and experimental pain. Pain *17*, 45-56.

Price, D.D., McHaffie, J.G., and Larson, M.A. (1989). Spatial summation of heat-induced pain: influence of stimulus area and spatial separation of stimuli on perceived pain sensation intensity and unpleasantness. J Neurophysiol *62*, 1270-1279.

Raehal, K.M., and Bohn, L.M. (2005). Mu opioid receptor regulation and opiate responsiveness. AAPS J *7*, E587-591.

Rainville, P. (2002). Brain mechanisms of pain affect and pain modulation. Curr Opin Neurobiol *12*, 195-204.

Rainville, P., Bao, Q.V., and Chretien, P. (2005). Pain-related emotions modulate experimental pain perception and autonomic responses. Pain *118*, 306-318.

Ramirez-Maestre, C., Esteve, R., and Lopez, A.E. (2008). Cognitive appraisal and coping in chronic pain patients. Eur J Pain *12*, 749-756.

Raynor, K., Kong, H., Chen, Y., Yasuda, K., Yu, L., Bell, G.I., and Reisine, T. (1994). Pharmacological characterization of the cloned kappa-, delta-, and mu-opioid receptors. Mol Pharmacol *45*, 330-334.

Rhudy, J.L., and Meagher, M.W. (2000). Fear and anxiety: divergent effects on human pain thresholds. Pain *84*, 65-75.

Rhudy, J.L., and Williams, A.E. (2005). Gender differences in pain: do emotions play a role? Gend Med *2*, 208-226.

Rhudy, J.L., Williams, A.E., McCabe, K.M., Rambo, P.L., and Russell, J.L. (2006). Emotional modulation of spinal nociception and pain: the impact of predictable noxious stimulation. Pain *126*, 221-233.

Rhudy, J.L., Williams, A.E., McCabe, K.M., Russell, J.L., and Maynard, L.J. (2008). Emotional control of nociceptive reactions (ECON): do affective valence and arousal play a role? Pain *136*, 250-261.

Ribeiro, S.C., Kennedy, S.E., Smith, Y.R., Stohler, C.S., and Zubieta, J.K. (2005). Interface of physical and emotional stress regulation through the endogenous opioid system and mu-opioid receptors. Prog Neuropsychopharmacol Biol Psychiatry *29*, 1264-1280.

Riley, J.L., Robinson, M.E., Wise, E.A., Myers, C.D., and Fillingim, R.B. (1998). Sex differences in the perception of noxious experimental stimuli: a meta-analysis. Pain *74*, 181-187.

Robinson, M.E., Gagnon, C.M., Riley, J.L., 3rd, and Price, D.D. (2003). Altering gender role expectations: effects on pain tolerance, pain threshold, and pain ratings. J Pain *4*, 284-288.

Robinson, M.E., Riley, J.L., 3rd, Myers, C.D., Papas, R.K., Wise, E.A., Waxenberg, L.B., and Fillingim, R.B. (2001). Gender role expectations of pain: relationship to sex differences in pain. J. Pain *2*, 251-257.

Robinson, M.E., and Wise, E.A. (2003). Gender bias in the observation of experimental pain. Pain *104*, 259-264.

Rolke, R., Baron, R., Maier, C., Tolle, T.R., Treede, R.D., Beyer, A., Binder, A., Birbaumer, N., Birklein, F., Botefur, I.C., *et al.* (2006a). Quantitative sensory testing in the German Research Network on Neuropathic Pain (DFNS): standardized protocol and reference values. Pain *123*, 231-243.

Rolke, R., Magerl, W., Campbell, K.A., Schalber, C., Caspari, S., Birklein, F., and Treede, R.D. (2006b). Quantitative sensory testing: a comprehensive protocol for clinical trials. Eur J Pain *10*, 77-88.

Rollman, G.B., Abdel-Shaheed, J., Gillespie, J.M., and Jones, K.S. (2004). Does past pain influence current pain: biological and psychosocial models of sex differences. Eur J Pain *8*, 427-433.

Roy, M., Peretz, I., and Rainville, P. (2008). Emotional valence contributes to music-induced analgesia. Pain *134*, 140-147.

Salomons, T.V., Johnstone, T., Backonja, M.M., and Davidson, R.J. (2004). Perceived controllability modulates the neural response to pain. J Neurosci *24*, 7199-7203.

Sarlani, E., Farooq, N., and Greenspan, J.D. (2003). Gender and laterality differences in thermosensation throughout the perceptible range. Pain *106*, 9-18.

Schaffner, N., Wittwer, A., Kut, E., Folkers, G., Benninger, D.H., and Candia, V. (2008). Heat pain threshold and tolerance show no left-right perceptual differences at complementary sites of the human forearm. Neurosci Lett *440*, 309-313.

Schiff, B.B., and Gagliese, L. (1994). The consequences of experimentally induced and chronic unilateral pain: reflections of hemispheric lateralization of emotion. Cortex *30*, 255-267.

Schiller, F. (1793). Ueber Anmuth und Würde (http://gutenberg.spiegel.de).

Schlereth, T., Baumgartner, U., Magerl, W., Stoeter, P., and Treede, R.D. (2003). Left-hemisphere dominance in early nociceptive processing in the human parasylvian cortex. Neuroimage *20*, 441-454.

Scott, D.J., Stohler, C.S., Egnatuk, C.M., Wang, H., Koeppe, R.A., and Zubieta, J.K. (2007). Individual differences in reward responding explain placebo-induced expectations and effects. Neuron *55*, 325-336.

Scott, D.J., Stohler, C.S., Egnatuk, C.M., Wang, H., Koeppe, R.A., and Zubieta, J.K. (2008). Placebo and nocebo effects are defined by opposite opioid and dopaminergic responses. Arch Gen Psychiatry *65*, 220-231.

Shy, M.E., Frohman, E.M., So, Y.T., Arezzo, J.C., Cornblath, D.R., Giuliani, M.J., Kincaid, J.C., Ochoa, J.L., Parry, G.J., and Weimer, L.H. (2003). Quantitative sensory testing: report of the Therapeutics and Technology Assessment Subcommittee of the American Academy of Neurology. Neurology *60*, 898-904.

Singer, T., Seymour, B., O'Doherty, J., Kaube, H., Dolan, R.J., and Frith, C.D. (2004). Empathy for Pain Involves the Affective but not Sensory Components of Pain. Science *303*, 1157-1162.

Singer, T., Seymour, B., O'Doherty, J.P., Stephan, K.E., Dolan, R.J., and Frith, C.D. (2006). Empathic neural responses are modulated by the perceived fairness of others. Nature *439*, 466-469.

Smith, Y.R., Stohler, C.S., Nichols, T.E., Bueller, J.A., Koeppe, R.A., and Zubieta, J.K. (2006). Pronociceptive and antinociceptive effects of estradiol through endogenous opioid neurotransmission in women. J Neurosci *26*, 5777-5785.

Spernal, J., Krieg, J.C., and Lautenbacher, S. (2003). Pain thresholds as a putative functional test for cerebral laterality in major depressive disorder and panic disorder. Neuropsychobiology *48*, 146-151.

Sprenger, T., Berthele, A., Platzer, S., Boecker, H., and Tolle, T.R. (2005). What to learn from in vivo opioidergic brain imaging? Eur J Pain *9*, 117-121.

Sprenger, T., Valet, M., Boecker, H., Henriksen, G., Spilker, M.E., Willoch, F., Wagner, K.J., Wester, H.J., and Tolle, T.R. (2006). Opioidergic activation in the medial pain system after heat pain. Pain.

Stefano, G.B., Salzet, B., and Fricchione, G.L. (1998). Enkelytin and opioid peptide association in invertebrates and vertebrates: immune activation and pain. Immunol Today *19*, 265-268.

Stein, C., and Mendl, G. (1988). The German counterpart to McGill Pain Questionnaire. Pain *32*, 251-255.

Steyer, R., Schwenkmezger, P., Notz, P., and Eid, M. (1997). Der Mehrdimensionale Befindlichkeitsfragebogen (MDBF). Handanweisung (Göttingen: Hogrefe).

Stich, S.P., and Warfield, T.A., eds. (2002). The Blackwell guide to philosophy of mind (Malden: Blackwell).

Stohler, C.S., and Kowalski, C.J. (1999). Spatial and temporal summation of sensory and affective dimensions of deep somatic pain. Pain *79*, 165-173.

Swanson, L.W. (2003). The amygdala and its place in the cerebral hemisphere. Ann N Y Acad Sci *985*, 174-184.

Symonds, L.L., Gordon, N.S., Bixby, J.C., and Mande, M.M. (2006). Right-lateralized pain processing in the human cortex: an FMRI study. J Neurophysiol *95*, 3823-3830.

Taylor, D.J., McGillis, S.L., and Greenspan, J.D. (1993). Body site variation of heat pain sensitivity. Somatosens Mot Res *10*, 455-465.

Thompson, E. (2007). Mind in life: biology, phenomenology, and the sciences of mind (Cambridge, Mass.: Harvard University Press).

Thorn, B.E., Clements K.L., Ward L.C., Dixon K.E., Kersh B.C., Boothby J.L., and W.F., C. (2004). Personality factors in the explanation of sex differences in pain catastrophizing and response to experimental pain. Clin. J. Pain *20*, 275-282.

Tracey, I., and Mantyh, P.W. (2007). The cerebral signature for pain perception and its modulation. Neuron *55*, 377-391.

Tracey, I., Ploghaus, A., Gati, J.S., Clare, S., Smith, S., Menon, R.S., and Matthews, P.M. (2002). Imaging attentional modulation of pain in the periaqueductal gray in humans. J Neurosci *22*, 2748-2752.

Treede, R.D., Meyer, R.A., and Campbell, J.N. (1990). Comparison of heat and mechanical receptive fields of cutaneous C-fiber nociceptors in monkey. J Neurophysiol *64*, 1502-1513.

Ulbrich, S. (2011). The Walking Tree - Organisation neuer Forschung in der Wissenschaft: Zusammenarbeit zwischen Integration und Differenzierung. Universität Magdebrug, Dissertation.

Valet, M., Sprenger, T., Boecker, H., Willoch, F., Rummeny, E., Conrad, B., Erhard, P., and Tolle, T.R. (2004). Distraction modulates connectivity of the cingulo-frontal cortex and the midbrain during pain--an fMRI analysis. Pain *109*, 399-408.

Veldhuijzen, D.S., Kenemans, J.L., de Bruin, C.M., Olivier, B., and Volkerts, E.R. (2006). Pain and attention: attentional disruption or distraction? J Pain *7*, 11-20.

Villemure, C., and Bushnell, M.C. (2002). Cognitive modulation of pain: how do attention and emotion influence pain processing? Pain *95*, 195-199.

Villemure, C., Slotnick, B.M., and Bushnell, M.C. (2003). Effects of odors on pain perception: deciphering the roles of emotion and attention. Pain *106*, 101-108.

Wager, T.D., Rilling, J.K., Smith, E.E., Sokolik, A., Casey, K.L., Davidson, R.J., Kosslyn, S.M., Rose, R.M., and Cohen, J.D. (2004). Placebo-induced changes in FMRI in the anticipation and experience of pain. Science *303*, 1162-1167.

Wasylak, T.J., Abbott, F.V., English, M.J., and Jeans, M.E. (1990). Reduction of postoperative morbidity following patient-controlled morphine. Can J Anaesth *37*, 726-731.

Weisenberg, M., Raz, T., and Hener, T. (1998). The influence of film-induced mood on pain perception. Pain *76*, 365-375.

Whipple, B., and Glynn, N.J. (1992). Quantification of the effects of listening to music as a noninvasive method of pain control. Sch Inq Nurs Pract *6*, 43-58; discussion 59-62.

Wiech, K., Farias, M., Kahane, G., Shackel, N., Tiede, W., and Tracey, I. (2008a). An fMRI study measuring analgesia enhanced by religion as a belief system. Pain *139*, 467-476.

Wiech, K., Ploner, M., and Tracey, I. (2008b). Neurocognitive aspects of pain perception. Trends Cogn Sci *12*, 306-313.

Wiech, K., and Tracey, I. (2009). The influence of negative emotions on pain: behavioral effects and neural mechanisms. Neuroimage.

Willer, J.C., Dehen, H., and Cambier, J. (1981). Stress-induced analgesia in humans: endogenous opioids and naloxone-reversible depression of pain reflexes. Science *212*, 689-691.

Willoch, F., Schindler, F., Wester, H.J., Empl, M., Straube, A., Schwaiger, M., Conrad, B., and Tolle, T.R. (2004). Central poststroke pain and reduced opioid receptor binding within pain processing circuitries: a [11C]diprenorphine PET study. Pain *108*, 213-220.

Woolf, V. (1926/2002). On being ill (Ashfield, MA: Paris Press).

Wunsch, A., Philippot, P., and Plaghki, L. (2003). Affective associative learning modifies the sensory perception of nociceptive stimuli without participant's awareness. Pain *102*, 27-38.

Yarnitsky, D., Simone, D.A., Dotson, R.M., Cline, M.A., and Ochoa, J.L. (1992). Single C nociceptor responses and psychophysical parameters of evoked pain: effect of rate of rise of heat stimuli in humans. J Physiol *450*, 581-592.

Yarnitsky, D., Sprecher, E., Zaslansky, R., and Hemli, J.A. (1995). Heat pain thresholds: normative data and repeatability. Pain *60*, 329-332.

Yosipovitch, G., Meredith, G., Chan, Y.H., and Goh, C.L. (2004). Do ethnicity and gender have an impact on pain thresholds in minor dermatologic procedures? A study on thermal pain perception thresholds in Asian ethinic groups. Skin. Res. Technol. *10*, 38-42.

Youell, P.D., Wise, R.G., Bentley, D.E., Dickinson, M.R., King, T.A., Tracey, I., and Jones, A.K. (2004). Lateralisation of nociceptive processing in the human brain: a functional magnetic resonance imaging study. Neuroimage *23*, 1068-1077.

Zadina, J.E., Hackler, L., Ge, L.J., and Kastin, A.J. (1997). A potent and selective endogenous agonist for the mu-opiate receptor. Nature *386*, 499-502.

Zeilhofer, H.U., Witschi, R., and Hosl, K. (2009). Subtype-selective GABAA receptor mimetics--novel antihyperalgesic agents? J Mol Med *87*, 465-469.

Zillmann, D., de Wied, M., King-Jablonski, C., and Jenzowsky, S. (1996). Drama-induced affect and pain sensitivity. Psychosom Med *58*, 333-341.

Zubieta, J.K., Bueller, J.A., Jackson, L.R., Scott, D.J., Xu, Y., Koeppe, R.A., Nichols, T.E., and Stohler, C.S. (2005). Placebo effects mediated by endogenous opioid activity on mu-opioid receptors. J Neurosci *25*, 7754-7762.

Zubieta, J.K., Ketter, T.A., Bueller, J.A., Xu, Y., Kilbourn, M.R., Young, E.A., and Koeppe, R.A. (2003). Regulation of human affective responses by anterior cingulate and limbic mu-opioid neurotransmission. Arch Gen Psychiatry *60*, 1145-1153.

Zubieta, J.K., Smith, Y.R., Bueller, J.A., Xu, Y., Kilbourn, M.R., Jewett, D.M., Meyer, C.R., Koeppe, R.A., and Stohler, C.S. (2001). Regional mu opioid receptor regulation of sensory and affective dimensions of pain. Science *293*, 311-315.

Zubieta, J.K., Smith, Y.R., Bueller, J.A., Xu, Y., Kilbourn, M.R., Jewett, D.M., Meyer, C.R., Koeppe, R.A., and Stohler, C.S. (2002). mu-opioid receptor-mediated antinociceptive responses differ in men and women. J Neurosci *22*, 5100-5107.

Zubieta, J.K., and Stohler, C.S. (2009). Neurobiological mechanisms of placebo responses. Ann N Y Acad Sci *1156*, 198-210.

Zyski, B., Bull, G., McDonald, W. & Johns, M. (1984). Perturbation analysis of normal and pathological larynges. Folia Phoniatr. *36*, 190-198.

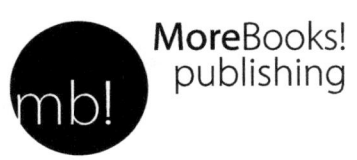
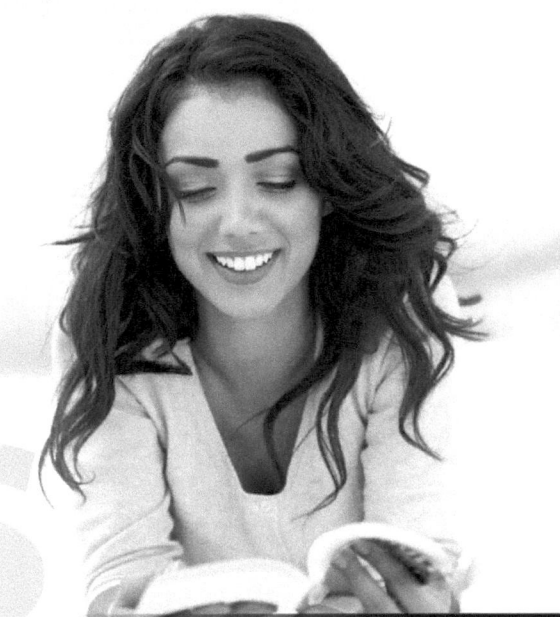

# i want morebooks!

Buy your books fast and straightforward online - at one of world's fastest growing online book stores! Environmentally sound due to Print-on-Demand technologies.

## Buy your books online at
### www.get-morebooks.com

Kaufen Sie Ihre Bücher schnell und unkompliziert online – auf einer der am schnellsten wachsenden Buchhandelsplattformen weltweit! Dank Print-On-Demand umwelt- und ressourcenschonend produziert.

## Bücher schneller online kaufen
### www.morebooks.de

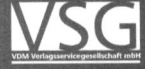

VDM Verlagsservicegesellschaft mbH
Heinrich-Böcking-Str. 6-8
D - 66121 Saarbrücken

Telefon: +49 681 3720 174
Telefax: +49 681 3720 1749

info@vdm-vsg.de
www.vdm-vsg.de

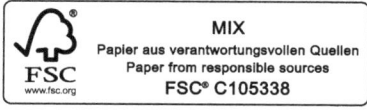

Printed by Books on Demand GmbH, Norderstedt / Germany